Best Methods For Treating Diabetes

M. K. Ansari, Ph.D.

RESEARCH PRESS

Research Press, New York

Notice to the reader:

Here is the health information you will find reliable; it has been drawn from the well reputed sources of latest science. However, this information is not meant to be a substitute for professional medical advice and care. The author and the publisher disclaim any or all liability arising from the application of any suggestion or information contained here. A health care professional should always be consulted regarding your specific situation.

Research Press, Inc., New York
94 Gardiners Ave, Suite 182
Levittown, NY 11756

Designed by Raheel Ansari
New York University School of Medicine

Printed in the United States of America

75 76 78 79 80 AT:08

ISBN 0-9765090-5-9

Library of Congress Cataloging-in-Publication Data

Ansari, M. K.
Best methods for treating diabetes / M.K.Ansari.
p. cm.
Includes bibliographical references and index.
ISBN 0-9765090-5-9 (pbk.)
1. Diabetes--Popular works. I. Title.
RC660.4.A547 2008
616.4'62--dc22

2008039762

Best Methods for Treating Diabetes

To my mother whose love I can't repay

Contents

Acknowledgments

Here are powerful methods of treating diabetes. They are drawn from the best of diabetes-science on the earth. I sincerely acknowledge the help I got from numerous precious resources, which enabled me present this empowering material.

Once again, as in the past, special thanks are due to Raheel Ansari, a talented, committed M.D. student of the New York University School of Medicine. He not only designed this book but also helped me in accessing the latest, cutting-edge medical literature on the subject.

1

Diabetes Treatment Plan

You will be diagnosed with diabetes when your blood sugar in a laboratory test matches any of the following blood sugar values:

Blood Sugar Values Representing Diabetes	
Type of Test	*Blood Sugar Value*
Fasting blood sugar	126 mg/dL (7.0 mmol/L) or greater
or	
Blood sugar 2 hours after drinking 75 grams of dry glucose mixed in water	200 mg/dL (11.1 mmol/L) or greater
or	
Casual/random blood sugar (with symptoms of diabetes such as excessive thirst, excessive urination, or weight loss)	200 mg/dL (11.1 mmol/L) or greater
Source: American Diabetes Association. American Association of Clinical Endocrinologists.	

Upon being diagnosed with diabetes, the immediate concern should be to control your blood sugar safely and keep it within the normal or near to normal range. This is necessary because uncontrolled diabetes heightens the risk for acute medical emergencies and long-term complications. Acute medical emergencies include low blood sugar (hypoglycemia), very high blood sugar (hyperosmolar hyperglycemic state), and increased acids in the blood (Diabetic ketoacidosis). These conditions are usually short-term and are corrected by timely treatment. However, delay in treating these medical emergencies can lead to serious consequences, including death.

Long-term complications of diabetes, on the other hand, result from long-standing uncontrolled blood sugar. Heart disease, stroke, kidney failure, blindness, amputation, and nerve pain are some of the common long-term complications.

You must control your blood sugar to protect yourself from diabetes complications. Your doctor will set your treatment goals and work out a treatment plan according to your individual needs and conditions. A treatment plan for diabetes has certain components:

SETTING A BLOOD SUGAR TARGET

The fist step in starting your diabetes treatment is to assess your condition and set a blood sugar target to be achieved. Your blood sugar target will be set according to treatment goals individualized for you. The table on the next page indicates usual targets of blood sugar for people with diabetes, and, as a comparison, it also shows desirable ranges of blood sugar for healthy people.

METHODS OF TREATMENT

After setting the blood sugar target, the next step is to choose a treatment method or methods to control your diabetes. Treatment methods include:

Blood Sugar Targets for Adults		
**Blood Sugar*	*Target for People with Diabetes*	*Target for People without Diabetes*
Fasting	90 to 130 mg/dL (5 to 7.2 mmol/L)	Less than 100 mg/dL (5.6 mmol/L)
After meals	Less than 180 mg/dL (10. 0 mmol/L)	Less than 110 mg/dL (6.1 mmol/L)
Bedtime	110 to 150 mg/dL (6.1 to 8.3 mmol/L)	Less than 120 mg/dL (6.6 mmol/L)
* As measured by a laboratory or tested on a glucose meter giving comparable results. (Most meters today give lab equivalent readings.)		
Source: American Diabetes Association. Joslin Diabetes Center.		

Healthy Lifestyle

A healthy lifestyle consisting of healthy eating, healthy weight, regular exercise, stop smoking, if you are a smoker, and managing your stress are essential elements in prevention and every treatment plan for diabetes.

Healthy Eating

Nutrition as a therapy helps control blood sugar. Good blood sugar control, in turn, helps prevent and manage diabetes related complications. In a healthy eating plan, you consume:

- Fiber rich foods such as whole-grain breads, bran cereals, brown rice, and beans.
- A variety of fruits and vegetables.
- Minimum possible amounts of saturated fat, trans fat, and cholesterol. Saturated fat is present in foods such as red meat and butter. Trans fat is present in most hamburgers, commercially fried and baked foods such as potato chips and cookies. Cholesterol- rich foods include organ meats, egg yolk, and butter.
- Low fat or fat free milk.
- Minimum amount of added sugars to make you able to eat more of other healthy foods. Foods with added sugar include sweetened syrups, regular soda drinks, sweetened fruit juices, cakes, candies, and cookies.
- Low to moderate amount of salt.
- Moderate amount of nuts (about 1/3 cup) 3 to 4 days a week. Nuts such as almonds, walnuts, and peanuts are good sources of monounsaturated fat, which is probably the healthiest type of all fats. Nuts may help control blood sugar.
- Moderate amount of alcohol if you choose to drink alcoholic beverages.

Regular Exercise

Exercise enhances the effect of your natural and injected insulin, leading to improved blood sugar control. In addition, with increase in effort and activity during exercise, the cells in your body pull in an increased amount of sugar from the blood, decreasing your raised blood sugar levels. Most people can include a moderate intensity physical activity such as brisk walking for at least 30 minutes every day in their exercise routine.

Healthy Weight

Excess body weight is a strong risk factor for type 2 diabetes. British and American studies are showing that excess weight may even accelerate the development of type 1 diabetes in young children and young adults. Aim for a healthy weight. A range between 18.5 to less than 25.0 in a weight measure known as BMI (body mass index) represents healthy weight. When you have excess weight and type 2 diabetes together, even a moderate weight loss will help control your blood sugar.

Stop Smoking

Tobacco smoking increases insulin resistance in the body, leading to raised blood sugar levels. Raised blood sugar tends to damage blood vessels throughout the body and heightens the risk for long-term complications of diabetes, including heart attack, stroke, and amputation. Stop smoking if you are a smoker; doing so will improve your blood sugar and reduce your risk for the long-term complications.

Managing Your Stress

Constant stress tends to produce insulin resistance in the body, which makes your blood sugar worse if you have type 2 diabetes. In addition, when stressed, you are likely to neglect your diet, exercise, medication, and self-monitoring of your blood sugar. As a result, you tend to lose control of your diabetes and are exposed to increased risks for long-term complications.

Manage your stress to help you keep healthy blood sugar levels. For managing the stress, learn how to relax, eat healthy, do not smoke, avoid or restrict alcohol intake, exercise regularly, take enough sleep, and spare some time for an enjoyable hobby. If necessary, take the help of a healthcare professional.

Medication

When healthy lifestyle measures fail to control blood sugar, drug treatment is added. Depending on the type of diabetes, its medical treatment may include any or a combination of the following aids:

- Diabetes pills.
- Injectable drugs such as pramlintide and exenatide.
- Insulin. It may be injected, inhaled, or continuously administered through an insulin pump. At present, however, insulin injections are the most common form of insulin delivery.

(More on diabetes medications, later.)

Pancreas Transplantation

In an extreme form of uncontrolled diabetes that does not respond even to intensive insulin treatment, pancreas or islet cell transplantation may be considered for people with type 1 diabetes (see title 14).

SELECTING THE METHOD OF TREATMENT

Treatment strategies for people with type 1 diabetes are different from those for people with type 2 diabetes. If you have type 1 diabetes, you must get insulin therapy. In type 1 diabetes, your pancreas stops producing insulin and you have no other option but to get insulin from outside the body such as through injections or through an insulin pump.

In type 2 diabetes, the treatment strategies range from lifestyle changes to insulin therapy. Upon diagnosis that you have type 2 diabetes, and unless drug treatment, including insulin, has become necessary, you should first adopt lifestyle changes to control your blood sugar. Planned meals, weight reduction if you carry excess body weight, increased physical activity, quitting tobacco smoking if you smoke, and managing stress will help control your blood sugar. You should try lifestyle changes at least for 6 months. When lifestyle changes fail to achieve your blood sugar goal, the doctor may decide to add diabetes pills, or other injectable drugs noted before, or insulin, or a combination of these drugs in your treatment plan. Healthy lifestyle, however, is the key component even when drug treatment is added.

As for treating gestational diabetes (diabetes occurring in pregnancy), diabetes pills are not recommended because of safety concerns. Gestational diabetes requires treatment with insulin (see title 12.4).

While setting your blood sugar target and choosing the treatment method to achieve it, safety and risk aspects of a treatment plan should always remain in consideration. Consult your doctor for help.

SELF-MONITORING OF BLOOD SUGAR

Self-testing of blood sugar and using the test results in management of diabetes is called self-monitoring of blood glucose (SMBG), which is an extremely useful tool in efficient management and treatment of diabetes. SMBG lets you know instantly the current status of your blood sugar: low, high, or within the target range. This knowledge allows you and your doctor to make quick treatment decisions, including adjustments in meals or snacks, exercise, and medication.

URINE KETONE TEST

High blood sugar, especially in people with type 1 diabetes, tends to increase poisonous acids (ketones) in the blood, causing increased excretion of ketones in the urine. This is a dangerous condition that can lead to coma and even death. If your SMBG consistently shows blood sugar, which is 300 mg/dL or greater, use a dipstick such as Chemstrip or Ketostix for testing the presence of ketones in urine. If the dipstick changes its color, it is a sign that ketones are present. Notify this condition to your doctor immediately.

A1C TEST

The glycosylated hemoglobin (A1C) test known as the A1C test shows how well your control of blood sugar has been during the last 2 to 3 months (see title 4). This test helps you monitor long-term control of your blood sugar, and guides you and your doctor in fine-tuning your treatment.

The present handbook, identifying the best methods for treating diabetes, will cover standard options and latest developments in the medical treatment of diabetes—diabetes pills, the newly developed injectable drugs, insulin injections, inhaled insulin, insulin pumps, and the extreme option of pancreas transplantation.

First, however, take a look at self-monitoring of blood sugar, the tool that will help you keep your treatment plan in track.

2

Self-Monitoring Your Blood Sugar

In a well-designed treatment plan of diabetes, self-monitoring of blood sugar is an essential part for making right treatment decisions. Self-monitoring of blood sugar or glucose (SMBG) guides you and your doctor to adjust and fine-tune your treatment plan, helping you reduce your risks for diabetes related complications.

METHODS OF SELF-MONITORING BLOOD SUGAR

At present, three methods of self-monitoring of blood sugar are available:

- Test strips read with reference to a color chart
- Test strips read by a glucose meter
- Automatic and continuous measuring device

In the test strip method, a small drop of blood is placed on a chemically saturated pad of a plastic strip. The chemical on the strip reacts with the blood drop and produces a color change, indicating the amount of sugar present in the blood. You can read this color change with reference to a color chart or use a glucose meter to read it. Blood sugar reading with reference to a color chart is less accurate than the reading made by a glucose meter.

The third method is to monitor blood sugar continuously. Several different kinds of continuous glucose monitoring systems are now available that automatically and continuously measure blood sugar around the clock. Some of these meters use a sensor, which inserted under the skin, measures blood sugar continuously and sends the measurements wirelessly to a receiver every 5 minutes or less.

Among the above three SMBG methods, reading of test stirps by a glucose meter is the most popular.

MEASURING BLOOD SUGAR ON GLUCOSE METERS

Using a glucose meter, you can self-monitor your blood sugar. This method of testing instantly measures how much your blood sugar is at the time of testing— normal, high, or low. The rapid results provided by this method of SMBG guide you to take timely action to correct low blood sugar; adjust your meals, medication, and physical activity to bring down raised blood sugar levels; or continue with the usual treatment if your blood sugar is within the target range. Testing blood sugar on glucose meters is an extremely useful tool that has revolutionized the management of diabetes.

SELF-MONITORING AND LABORATORY TESTING

In self-monitoring your blood sugar, using the the test strip method, you draw a drop of blood directly from a blood capillary (very small blood vessel) by piercing a lancet usually in your finger. This is a whole blood sample that contains red blood cells. Home glucose meters use whole blood samples on the test strips to measure blood sugar. Laboratory equipment, on the other hand, removes blood cells from a blood sample drawn from a vein, leaving behind a clear yellowish fluid part of the blood called plasma. Laboratories measure sugar in plasma blood. Because sugar gets concentrated in the plasma, the plasma-based blood sugar results are about 12 percent higher than the results given by your glucose meter that uses the whole blood sample.

Most glucose meters, today, reference their results with the laboratory results. This means that the results given by the plasma-calibrated glucose meters will almost be the same as those reported by the laboratories.

FREQUENCY OF TESTING

How often should you test your blood sugar? Your doctor will advise you how many times you should do it, depending on your treatment goals. However, general medical guidelines are:

- If you take 3 or more injections of insulin per day or use an insulin pump for constant infusion of insulin (intensive insulin therapy), self-monitor your blood sugar at least four times daily: once before each meal (breakfast, lunch, and dinner), and once at bedtime. The pre-meal testing will guide you as to how much insulin you should take to cover the after-meal rise of blood sugar. Bedtime testing, on the other hand, will help you cover the night: take an additional dose of insulin if your blood sugar is high or eat a snack if it is low.
- If you tend to have low blood sugar without symptoms, or frequently experience its symptoms, test your blood sugar more often.
- People with diabetes, when ill, should check their blood sugar more frequently. During your sick days, insulin becomes less efficient, resulting in poor control of blood sugar. By testing your blood sugar frequently when you are sick, you can appropriately adjust your dose of insulin or diabetes pills for better control of blood sugar.
- Test more frequently during pregnancy.

to exercise. This is necessary because if you start exercising with high or low blood sugar, your blood sugar may rise or fall to risky levels.

- If you are making changes in your physical activity, food intake, or diabetes medication, you should do some extra checking of your blood sugar.
- Test your blood sugar before you drive, especially when you are taking insulin or the sulfonylurea class of drugs to control blood sugar. Using these drugs may increase the risk for low blood sugar.
- If you have type 2 diabetes and it remains well controlled by using diabetes pills, you may test your blood sugar twice a week.
- Test your blood sugar whenever you experience any unusual symptoms.

SMBG RECORD KEEPING

Every time you test your blood sugar, write down the results in a diary or a log book. Compare these results with your blood sugar goal. You should also know how to handle situations when your SMBG results are higher or lower than your target, and what adjustments you should make in your diet, activity, and medication to achieve the target range. When your SMBG results repeatedly show poor blood sugar control, discuss the results with your doctor. The SMBG record will greatly help the doctor in making right treatment decisions for you. Your diary can become even more useful when now and then you also note down what and when you ate, how much you exercised, the type and dosage of the diabetes medication you took, and any stress you had.

Your health care professional should periodically check your monitoring technique to make sure that your meter readings are accurate and your method of checking is correct.

3

Glucose Meters

Glucose meters of a large variety are available today in the market. The prevailing trend in these meters is to make them less painful, more user friendly, and innovative. Glucose meters, because of their convenience of use and rapidity of results, are now commonly used for routine testing in hospitals also. The recent advancements in the meter technology have made the present day glucose meters more advanced and more accurate than before. Some glucose meters are basic; others are more advanced. Basic meters have fewer features, whereas the advanced meters come with a greater number of features.Your doctor or a diabetes educator will guide you in selecting a glucose meter that is right for you. Here are some important features of the glucose meters:

Test Memory

A glucose meter may or may not have a memory to store blood sugar test results. Some meters may store one past test result, whereas others may store in memory as many as 1,000 or even 4,000 past test results.

Test Time

Glucose meters, depending on their design, take varying times to display blood sugar readings: 5, 8, 10, 15, 20, 25, 30, 45, or 60 seconds.

Plasma Calibrated Values

Although glucose meters use whole blood to measure blood sugar, newer meters express their test results referenced with plasma blood. These readings are comparable with laboratory results. Some meters, however, still express readings referenced with whole blood values. Both methods are correct. As noted before, blood sugar results expressed in plasma blood values are about 12 percent greater than the blood sugar numbers referenced with whole blood values.

Size of Blood Sample

Some meters require a blood drop about the size of a pinhead; others use larger drops.

Data Port

Another feature that is becoming increasingly common in glucose meters is the provision of a data port. A data port in the meter allows it to work with diabetes management software in which you can transfer the information stored in the memory of the meter to a computer. The computer uses this information to display graphs, charts, and reports of your past test results. This feature may be helpful to your doctor in fine-tuning your treatment. In general, however, the usefulness of this feature has not been established.

Averaging of Test Results

Some glucose meters have the capability of averaging your blood sugar test results for the last several days to several weeks. A test average may give you an idea how good or bad your blood sugar control has been during the given period. This knowledge can help you and your doctor in adjusting your treatment.

Maintenance

Some glucose meters need regular internal cleaning, whereas others do not.

Multiple Tests

A few meters, using separate test strips can run multiple blood tests for sugar, cholesterol, triglycerides, and ketones at one platform.

Sites Other Than Fingertips

Some meters allow you to take blood samples from sites other than the fingertips. The alternate sites include the upper side of the forearm, upper arm, abdomen, and leg, where there are fewer nerve-endings that make the testing less painful. However, in certain conditions such as after you have eaten a meal or taken an insulin dose or have exercised, the blood sample taken from your fingertip will show changes in your blood sugar more quickly than a sample taken from other sites of your body such as the arm.

Audio Meter

"Talking" glucose meters are available that may be helpful for people who have sight problems. Theses are audio meters, which guide the user step-by-step through testing.

Test Strips

Some meters use easy-to-handle test strips. These include touchable test strips; touching their test areas has no effect on the test results. In some test strips, you can add more blood on the same strip during testing if the blood drop is not enough.

Lancet

To self-test your blood sugar, you pierce a lancet or needle in your finger tip or other sites of the body to draw a blood sample. Most people use a lancing device (a pen-like holder) that holds a lancet in place and pierces the skin. A laser device is also available, which uses a laser beam rather than a steel lancet to obtain a blood sample without pain.

However, the lancet is the most commonly used device in drawing blood samples in self-monitoring of blood sugar. Follow the instructions of the meter's manufacturer in drawing a blood sample. In general, rub your finger to warm it up for easy blood flow. (It can be any finger you feel comfortable with, but rotate the fingers or sites in the same finger in successive tests.) Clean the finger site with an alcohol swab. Let the site be dry. Pierce the lancet and squeeze the site slightly for getting a drop of blood for testing.

4

Hemoglobin A1C

The hemoglobin A1C test, also known as HbA1c, is a blood test that shows the average amount of your blood sugar during the last 2 to 3 months. The main purpose of this test is to monitor how well your blood sugar control has been over the last 2 to 3 months (poor control of diabetes for a prolonged period heightens the risk of organ damage, organ failure, or organ loss.) The A1C test helps predict and prevent diabetes complications from raised blood sugar.

How the Test Works

The hemoglobin A1C test is based on the interaction sugar has with hemoglobin. Hemoglobin (Hb) is a protein inside the red blood cells, transporting oxygen throughout the body. As the blood circulates in your body, sugar tends to stick to hemoglobin, a process called glycosylation. When you do not have diabetes, sugar sticks to about 5 percent of your hemoglobin. But in the presence of diabetes, when sugar is high in the blood, the amount of sugar attaching to the hemoglobin also increases. Once sugar is attached to hemoglobin, it remains there until the life span of the hemoglobin-containing red blood cell. (The life span of a red blood cell is about 2 to 3 months; old red blood cells are replaced by new red blood cells.) Because the A1C test measures the amount of sugar attached to hemoglobin in the red blood cells, the test also shows the average of your blood sugar relating to this period (2 to 3 months).

Although the A1C test measures blood sugar changes during the last 2 to 3 months, it is affected very much by the changes in blood sugar during the 1 month period preceding the test. Because the A1C test is affected more by the recent rather than the earlier changes in blood sugar, it can detect the effect of changes you made in your diet, exercise, and medication within the prior 2 to 3 weeks.

A1C Test Results

A1C test results indicate the percentage of hemoglobin that has been glycosylated in the blood (affected by sugar). Laboratories may adopt different ranges for normal values; check what is the normal range adopted by the laboratory doing your A1C test. Here is how th the American Diabetes Association (ADA) classifies A1C test results:

Less than 6 percent	Normal
Less than 7 percent	Goal for people with diabetes. In individual cases, the goal of less than 6 percent may be considered for people with diabetes and for pregnant people, if doing so is safe.
Greater than 8 percent	Needs intensive treatment.

Implications of A1C

Because raised levels of A1C mean raised levels of blood sugar for a prolonged period, such levels are strongly associated with the risk for long-term organ damage from diabetes. An A1C value above 9.5 percent is an indicator of very poor control of blood sugar, which is highly risky. Raised A1C levels call for aggressive management of diabetes. Research shows that if you control your blood sugar and lower your raised A1C level by even a small amount, you can improve your chances of living a healthy life. When you keep your A1C level below 7 percent, you can significantly reduce your risk for long-term damage from diabetes.

A1C Test, How Often?

The ADA suggests A1C testing at least twice a year for people with diabetes whose blood sugar is well controlled. As for people whose blood sugar is poorly controlled or who have changed their treatment plan, the ADA recommends A1C testing every 3 months for close monitoring.

Comparing the A1C Values

The A1C test results are expressed in percentages. To have an idea how these percentages compare with the average levels of your blood sugar, here is the conversion table:

A1C Conversion Values

A1C (%)	*Average Blood Sugar* * *(mg/dL)*	*mmol/L*
5	100	5.5
6	135	7.5
7	170	9.5
8	205	11.5

* Blood sugar values as measured by a laboratory or comparable results displayed by glucose meters referenced with the lab test.

Note: Each 35 mg/dL (2 mmol/L) increase in blood sugar raises your A1C level by 1 percent.

The A1C test is usually done by a laboratory. However, now tests are also available in which you collect a "fingerstick" blood sample, place it on a special collection card to dry, and mail it to a designated lab for processing. Disposable one-time test kits for home use have also come. These tests, using a blood sample from the fingertip, allow you to self-measure your A1C level. Blood samples for testing A1C can be drawn any time, even immediately after a meal.

Because A1C test is an indicator of average blood sugar over a period, and not the actual blood sugar at the time of testing, experts do not recommend it for the initial diagnosis of diabetes.

FRUCTOSAMINE TEST

This is a blood test usually done in a laboratory; it indicates your blood sugar control over the past 2 to 3 weeks. The fructosamine test is somewhere in between the daily SMBG that shows your blood sugar level at the time of testing, and the A1C test that shows the average of blood sugar over the past 2 to 3 months.

The basic principle of the fructosamine test is similar to the A1C test: sugar tends to attach with proteins during blood circulation. The A1C test measures the amount of sugar attaching to hemoglobin (protein), whereas the fructosamine test measures sugar that attaches to all other proteins in the blood, mainly albumin. Because most proteins (except hemoglobin) last in the blood for only about 2 to 3 weeks, the fructosamine test shows the average of blood sugar during the last 2 to 3 week period. Since this test detects changes of blood sugar control within weeks, rather than months, it may be more useful than the A1C test in making treatment adjustments in such conditions as pregnancy.

The fructosamine test, though, may have a place in the monitoring of your blood sugar; it cannot replace self-monitoring and the A1C. Regular self-monitoring of blood sugar as suggested by your doctor, and testing hemoglobin A1C every 3 months, are major tools for monitoring your blood sugar and making necessary treatment decisions to control diabetes.

5

Diabetes Pills

Diabetes pills, also called oral hypoglycemic agents (OHA), are drugs taken by mouth to lower blood sugar. These pills work by interacting with natural insulin in the body and are given to a person with type 2 diabetes in whom the pancreas is still producing at least some insulin. Diabetes pills will not work if you have type 1 diabetes and your pancreas has stopped producing insulin.

TYPES OF DIABETES PILLS

At present, six different classes of pills are available to treat type 2 diabetes:

- Sulfonylurea
- Biguanide (metformin)
- Alpha-glucosidase inhibitor
- Thiazolidinedione
- Meglitinide
- DPP-4 inhibitor

The following reviews will look at the broad features of these blood sugar lowering-agents. The brand-named diabetes pills referred to in these reviews are those currently available in the United States. Each class of these pills lowers blood sugar in its own different way.

5.1

Sulfonylureas

Sulfonylurea is the oldest class of diabetes medicine to lower blood sugar. The pills in this class are usually the first line of drugs used in treatment of type 2 diabetes. Here are the key features of these pills:

SULFONYLUREA

Sulfonylurea: First Generation

Generic name	*Brand name*	*Dose (mg per day)*
Chlorpropamide	Diabinese	100 to 500

Sulfonylureas: Second Generation

Generic name	*Brand name*	*Dose (mg per day)*
Glimepiride	Amaryl	1.0 to 4
Glipizide	Glucotrol	2.5 to 40
Glipizide-GITS	Glucotrol-XL	2.5 to 20
Glyburide	Micronase	2.5 to 20
	DiaBeta	2.5 to 20
	Glynase Pres	1.5 to 12

Note: Tolazamide (Tolinase) and tolbutamide (Orinase) have been discontinued.

How the drug works

The principal action of sulfonylureas is to stimulate secretion of insulin from the pancreas. Their secondary actions are to increase body's response to insulin, and reduce production of sugar by the liver. All these effects lead to lowering of blood sugar.

Important facts about the drug:

- Sulfonylureas are especially useful for controlling blood sugar in thin people with type 2 diabetes who fail to control blood sugar by diet alone.
- When sulfonylureas are used alone to treat high blood sugar, they lower hemoglobin A1C by about 1 to 2 percent.
- The effectiveness of this class of drug varies with individuals: some people may never achieve full control of blood sugar or many lose control after its prolonged use.
- When a single dose of a sulfonylurea does not lower blood sugar to the desired target, dividing the dose and taking these doses in the morning and evening may help.
- When sulfonylureas alone are ineffective in achieving good blood sugar control, drugs from the other class or classes may be added.
- A study published in 2003 in the *Journal of the American College of Cardiology* suggests that sulfonylureas such as glyburide or glipizide mask the severity of heart attacks. When a person is having a severe heart attack, and he or she has been using the sulfonylurea class of pills to control blood sugar, the EKG may not indicate the true electrical changes in the heart. As a result, such a person may not get proper treatment.

Risk of low blood sugar

Sulfonylurea drugs can cause a severe fall in blood sugar, especially when you take this class of drug, and skip a meal, or exercise vigorously.

Effect on blood fats

These drugs do not improve cholesterol and other blood fats.

Effect on weight

It may increase weight.

Main side effect

Low blood sugar.

Other possible side effects

Stomach pain and itching.

Caution

This drug is not for you if you ever experienced reaction with sulfa drugs in the past.

5.2

Biguanide (Metformin)

The only medicine in the biguanide class is metformin. Here are its key features:

BIGUANIDE

Generic name	*Brand name*	*Dose (mg per day)*
Metformin	Glucophage	500 to 2,550
	Glucophage XR	500 to 2,000

How the drug works

The principal action of metformin is to reduce the amount of sugar released by your liver. Second, it decreases insulin resistance in the body. Both these effects lower blood sugar.

Important facts about the drug:

- Metformin, when used alone, is as effective as the sulfonylureas are in the long term.
- Metformin is often added with other classes of diabetes

pills and insulin, and because it works in a different way, it has an additive effect in lowering blood sugar.

- It is useful in obese patients with cholesterol and other blood fat disorders.

Risk of low blood sugar

Metformin by itself does not cause low blood sugar.

Effect on blood fats

Metformin decreases raised triglyceride levels.

Effect on weight

It does not increase weight; actually, it may lead to some weight loss.

Main side effect

High levels of metformin in the blood may raise lactic acid levels in the blood, a condition called lactic acidosis. Lactic acidosis may lead to severe fatigue, unusual muscle pain, irregular heartbeats, difficulty breathing, unusual abdominal discomfort, dizziness, shallow breathing, and sleepiness that may turn into a coma. Because of the potential risk of lactic acidosis, people who use metformin are advised to stop metformin usually 48 hours before having a surgery.

Other possible side effects

Lack of appetite, weight loss, diarrhea, and metallic taste in the mouth.

Caution. Metformin is not recommended for people with active kidney and liver diseases and heart failure.

METFORMIN MIXTURES

In the United States, combination pills for lowering blood sugar in type 2 diabetes mostly include metformin mixed with other oral agents (see table below). The mixtures combine the effects of the mixed drugs.

Metformin "Mixed" Pills		
Generic name	*Brand name*	*Dose (mg per day)*
glyburide plus metmormin	Glucovance	1.25/250 to 20/2000
glipizide plus metformin	Metaglip	2.5/250 to 20/2,000
rosiglitazone plus metformin	Avandamet	4/1, 000 to 8/2,000
rosiglitazone plus glimepiride	Avandaryl	4/2 to 8/4
pioglitazone plus metformin	Actosplus Met	15/500 to 45/2,550
sitagliptin plus metformin	Janumet	50/1,000 to 100/2,000
Source: *Epocrates Drug Reference*.2007.		

5·3

Alpha-Glucosidase Inhibitors

Here are the key features of this class of diabetes pills:

ALPHA-GLUCOSIDASE INHIBITORS

Generic name	*Brand name*	*Dose (mg per day)*
Acarbose	Precose	25 to 300
Miglitol	Glyset	25 to 300

Note: Acarbose is the popular medicine in this class.

How the drug works

Acarbose temporarily blocks the activity of digestive enzymes, and delays digestion of food. Slow absorption of food into the body leads to slow rise of blood sugar after eating meals.

Important facts about the drug

- Because acarbose delays absorption of food in the blood, it is sometimes preferred for people who usually experience rapid rise of blood sugar after meals.
- Acarbose is taken just before the first bite of the main meals.

- When used alone, acarbose is not as good as sulfonylurea and metformin are in controlling blood sugar in the long term.
- Acarbose is often combined with other classes of diabetes pills to achieve better control of blood sugar.
- When you add diabetes pills of other class or classes to acarbose, be careful that your blood sugar does not drop too low. To treat low blood sugar, take oral glucose (dextrose) that is quickly absorbed in the blood. Table sugar or starches, because of their relatively more complex chemical structure than dextrose, may not work quickly since acarbose slows down their absorption in the body.

Risk of low blood sugar

Acarbose by itself does not cause low blood sugar.

Effect on blood fats

It slightly improves blood fats.

Effect on weight

It does not increase weight.

Main side effects

Gas, abdominal pain, bloating, and diarrhea, conditions that may settle down over time.

Other possible side effects

Nausea, fatigue, and headache.

Caution

Acarbose is not recommended in the presence of active liver diseases or any intestinal and digestive problems, including inflammatory bowel disease.

5·4

Thiazolidinediones (TZDs)

This is a new class of diabetes pills. Here are its key features:

THIAZOLIDINEDIONES (TZDs)

Generic name	*Brand name*	*Dose (mg per day)*
Pioglitazone	Actos	15 to 45
Rosiglitazone	Avandia	2 to 8

How the drug works

The primary function of thiazolidinediones (TZDs) is to increase your body's sensitivity to insulin, which in turn enhances the action of your own insulin in the body. Second, TZDs reduce production of sugar by the liver. Both these effects help lower blood sugar. This drug does not stimulate secretion of insulin from the pancreas.

Important facts about the drug

- Thiazolidinediones are useful in people having insulin resistance.

- Generally, these drugs are not used alone; they are added to other classes of diabetes pills or insulin.
- Thiazolidinediones are not better than sulfonylureas or metformin in reducing blood sugar on a long-term basis.
- TZDs may decrease the effect of birth control pills.
- These drugs may take several weeks before they start working.
- TZDs may affect the liver. You should have a blood test (liver function test) every 2 months during the first year of treatment with these drugs, and periodically thereafter for monitoring the function of your liver.

Risk of low blood sugar

Thiazolidinediones alone do not cause low blood sugar.

Effect on blood fats

The effect varies. This drug may increase total blood cholesterol and LDL cholesterol, and decrease triglycerides.

Effect on weight

It increases weight.

Main side effect

Water retention in the body, causing swelling in the legs and ankles and unusual weakness and tiredness.

Other possible side effects

Difficulty breathing, swelling of the lips, tongue, or face, hives, nausea, vomiting, abdominal pain, loss of appetite, unusual fatigue, and yellowing of the skin.

Caution

Rezulin (troglitazone), a drug of the thiazolidinedione class manufactured by Parke-Davis was withdrawn from the market in March 2000 on the reports that several people died from liver failure due to liver damage caused by this drug. Another bad report in 2007: research has raised safety concerns about another diabetes pill in this class —Avandia (rosiglitazone). Medical journals have reported a disturbing finding that Avandia, the widely used pill to treat type 2 diabetes, may increase the chances of having a heart attack in some patients. However, as of today, the US health experts have not recommended to discontinue this drug, but insist, that it should be used very cautiously.

Thiazolidinediones are linked to causing buildup of excess water in the body (water retention). People who already have this problem due to heart disease should be cautious while using these drugs.

5·5

Meglitinide

Here are the key features of diabetes pills in this class.

MEGLITINIDE

Generic name	*Brand name*	*Dose (mg per day)*
Repaglinide	Prandin	0.5 to 16
Nateglinide	Starlix	60 to 360

How the drug works

Meglitinide has a different chemical composition from sulfonylurea, but its effect is similar: it lowers blood sugar by stimulating insulin secretion from the pancreas right after meals.

Important facts about the drug

- Meglitinide is quick in action but short in duration. It is rapidly absorbed in the blood within 20 minutes, and peaks its action in about 1 hour after you have taken the pill. Meglitinide is usually used for controlling the after-meal rise of blood sugar. If your problem is a rapid rise in blood sugar after meals (postprandial sugar) rather than blood sugar in the fasting state, your doctor may prescribe this drug.

- It is useful for people with type 2 diabetes, having irregular meal patterns. You take this drug when you take a meal, and miss it when you skip the meal.
- This drug is taken about 20 to 30 minutes before a meal.
- It may be used alone or combined with metformin.

Risk of low blood sugar

The drug may cause low blood sugar.

Effect on blood fats

No effect.

Effect on weight

It increases weight.

Main side effect

Low blood sugar.

Other possible side effects

Cold and flu-like symptoms, joint aches, back pain, upset stomach, and dizziness.

Caution

Meglitinide is not recommended if you experienced allergy to this drug before, or your liver is seriously sick.

6

Novel Drugs for Lowering Blood Sugar

Novel drugs have been introduced, which lower blood sugar by influencing hormones in the intestines. These drugs work on the principle that when you eat food, intestinal hormones called incretins are produced in your gastrointestinal tract. These hormones help control your blood sugar by:

- Increasing secretion of insulin.
- Slowing down movement of food in the stomach, thereby delaying the speed at which sugar enters the bloodstream.
- Making you feel full, eat less, and lose weight.

However, these hormones (especially the two main incretins called GLP-1 and GIP) produced after a meal, are low in people with type 2 diabetes. The new drugs, targeting these incretins in circulation, boost and prolong their activity, leading to improved blood sugar control in people with type 2 diabetes.

At present, two incretin-influencing drugs — sitagliptin (brand name: Januvia), and injectable exenatide (brand name:Byetta)— have been approved by the U.S. Food and Drug Administration (FDA) for lowering blood sugar in people with type 2 diabetes.

The FDA has approved one more new drug, pramlintide

(brand name: Symlin), an injectable drug for treating both type 1 and type 2 diabetes. This drug is a synthetic form of human amylin, a naturally occurring hormone that along with insulin is produced in the beta cells of the pancreas and helps control blood sugar. In people with type 2 diabetes who use insulin and in people with type 1 diabetes, secretion of both insulin and amylin decreases. Injecting pramlintide improves this condition and leads to improved control of blood sugar after meals.

The next three titles contain more information about these novel blood sugar- lowering agents.

6.1

Sitagliptin

Sitagliptin (brand name: Januvia) is a new class of drug, which influences your intestinal hormones to lower blood sugar. This medicine is for adults with type 2 diabetes who do not take insulin to control blood sugar.

How the drug works

Sitagliptin, blocking an insulin-unfriendly enzyme called DPP-4, regulates the levels of insulin your body produces after eating. Regulated insulin levels help control blood sugar when it is high. It also decreases the amount of sugar produced by the liver.

Important facts about the drug

- Sitagliptin is taken once a day, at any time of the day.
- It lowers blood sugar immediately after a meal and between the meals.
- Sitagliptin does not lower your blood sugar when it is at healthy level or low; it works only when your blood sugar is high.
- You can use sitagliptin alone or in combination with metformin or TZD class of diabetes pills.
- Do not use it in children without the advice of the doctor.
- Sitagliptin is not for people with type 1 diabetes whose bodies have stopped producing insulin.

Risk of low blood sugar

Sitagliptin by itself does not cause low blood sugar.

Effect on blood fats

It does not increase or decrease blood fat levels.

Effect on weight

It does not increase weight.

Main side effects

Throat and lung infections; sore throat; and headache.

Other possible side effects

Nausea, diarrhea, abdominal pain, urinary tract infections, and allergic reactions such as swelling on the face and rash.

Dose

The usual recommended dose of sitagliptin is 100 mg once daily, either alone or in combination with metformin or TZDs.

Caution

The dose of sitagliptin needs to be reduced in people with moderate to severe kidney disease, including people receiving dialysis. The doctor may reduce the dose to 50 or 25 mg, depending on the severity of kidney disease.

6.2

Exenatide

Exenatide, brand name: Byetta, is an injectable drug for lowering blood sugar in people with type 2 diabetes. It is the first drug in a class known as incretin mimetics. Incretin mimetic is a drug that mimics the action of intestinal hormones called incretins.

How the drug works

Exenatide mimics blood sugar-lowering actions of incretins:

- It suppresses production of sugar from the liver.
- It slows down movement of food in the stomach, leading to delayed stomach emptying and slow absorption of sugar in the blood.
- It reduces appetite.
- It helps preserve the function of insulin producing cells in the pancreas.

All these actions lead to improved blood sugar control.

Important facts about the drug:

- Exenatide is a man-made version of a natural compound in the saliva of the Gila monster lizard. Gila monster lizard is a highly poisonous lizard of the southwestern United States and Mexico. It is named after the Gila River Basin of the southwestern United States.

- It is not a substitute for insulin in people with diabetes whose diabetes requires insulin treatment. Exenatide is not meant for people with type 1 diabetes.
- It improves blood sugar both in the fasting state and after meals.
- It stimulates insulin release from the pancreas when your blood sugar is high; it does not not lower blood sugar when it is already low.
- People with type 2 diabetes who have not been able to achieve desirable blood sugar control while using other diabetes pills may add exenatide in their treatment plan.
- Use of exenatide with insulin has not been studied.
- Exenatide (Byetta) is available in the form of prefilled pens in 5 mcg and 10 mcg per dose strengths. Each pen contains 60 doses.
- Once used, the pen should be discarded after 30 days. Exenatide, whether unopened or in use, should be kept in a refrigerator (not in the freezer).

Risk of low blood sugar

Risk for low blood sugar does not increase when metformin is included in the treatment with exenatide. The risk, however, becomes mild to moderate when exenatide and a medicine from the sulfonylurea class are combined.

Effect on blood fats

Treatment with exenatide leads to a small decrease in total cholesterol and LDL (bad) cholesterol. It has been shown to decrease triglyceride by about 37 mg/dL, and increase HDL(good) cholesterol by 4.5 mg/dL approximately.

Effect on weight

It reduces weight.

Main side effects

Nausea. People may experience nausea at the beginning of treatment; its frequency and severity decreases with continued therapy in most people.

Other possible side effects

Tiredness and decreased appetite.

Dose

The initial dose of exenatide is 5 mcg twice daily administered at any time within 60 minute before the morning and evening meals. (Exenatide should not be injected after a meal.) After 1 month of treatment, the dose of exenatide may be increased to 10 mcg twice daily. When exenatide is added to a sulfonylurea, the dose of the sulfonylurea may be reduced to decrease the risk of low blood sugar.

Caution

Exenatide is not recommended for people with severe kidney disease or those receiving dialysis. Pregnant people who plan to use exenatide should do so only after consulting their doctor. See recent warning from the Food and Drug Administration (FDA):

WARNING

The FDA received reports about the occurrence of acute pancreatitis in some patients from the use of Byetta. Pancreatitis is severe inflammation of the pancreas, a condition that can be life-threatening.

Although the FDA has not advised discontinuation of Byetta, it suggests that if people treated with this drug experience an unexplained abdominal pain with or without vomiting, they should quickly report this condition to their doctors. If the doctor diagnoses acute pancreatitis due to Byetta (and not due to other factors such as drinking too much alcohol and the presence of gallstones), the FDA suggests to discontinue the drug and not restart it.

6.3

Pramlintide

Pramlintide, brand name: Symlin, is a new injectable drug to lower blood sugar. It is meant for adults with type 1 and type 2 diabetes who already take insulin but have failed to achieve desired blood sugar control. Pramlintide, when added to mealtime insulin therapy, helps control blood sugar, especially after eating meals.

How the drug works

As you inject pramlintide and insulin at the time you eat meals, both the drugs work together to control blood sugar. Here is how it works. After you eat food, pramlintide slows down its movement into the stomach, which, in turn, slows down the speed at which sugar produced from the digested food enters the bloodstream. When sugar enters the blood, the injected insulin moves it into the tissues. Thus, pramlintide and insulin, working together, help prevent rapid peaks of blood sugar after eating, and stabilize blood sugar control.

Important facts about the drug:

- Pramlintide is injected immediately before each major meal containing at least 250 calories or at least 30 grams of carbohydrate.
- You will inject pramlintide with the insulin you take at meal times such as regular or rapid-acting insulin. Pramlintide works with mealtime insulin.

- Do not mix pramlintide and insulin in the same syringe, because insulin may affect pramlintide when the two are mixed together.
- When you take pramlintide, you may need to cut your insulin dose by 50 percent.
- Like insulin, inject pramlintide under the skin of your upper arm, abdomen, or thighs.
- You should frequently test your blood sugar— before and after every meal and at bedtime— when you take pramlintide.
- Because pramlintide slows the movement of food in the stomach, do not take it with other diabetes pills of similar action such as acarbose and miglitol. Taking these drugs together may cause a severe fall in your blood sugar.

Risk of low blood sugar

Blood sugar may fall too low, especially in people with type 1 diabetes. Low blood sugar may occur within 3 hours following a pramlintide injection.

Effect on blood fats

No effect.

Effect on weight

Pramlintide promotes feeling of fullness at meals, which, in turn, helps you lose weight.

Main side effect

The main side effect is nausea, which is high at the beginning of treatment, but decreases with time in most people. Nearly 9 percent of people taking pramlintide discontinued it because of nausea.

Other possible side effects

These include abdominal pain, decreased appetite, tiredness, and minor bruises at the site of injecting the drug.

Caution

Do not take pramlintide injection if:

- You cannot recognize symptoms of low blood sugar, a condition called low blood sugar unawareness.
- You have a stomach problem called gastroparesis in which food takes too long to pass through the stomach.
- You do not plan to eat food for any reason.
- You are pregnant or breast-feeding and have not consulted your doctor.

If you inject pramlintide in the above conditions, your blood sugar may drop to dangerously low levels.

Dose

Unlike insulin that is measured in units, pramlintide dose is measured in micrograms (mcg). However, most common doses of pramlintide are equivalent to insulin doses in a syringe:

Pramlintide dose (mcg)	*U-100 Insulin syringe units*
15	2.5
30	5.0
45	7.5
60	10
120	20

As for dosage of pramlintide, note:

- The initial dose is 60 mcg for people with type 2 diabetes, and 15 mcg for people with type 1 diabetes, immediately before a major meal.
- Reduce your dose of premeal insulin (including rapid acting, short acting, 70/30 or 75/25 by 50 percent) while injecting pramlintide.
- If no significant nausea or low blood sugar occurs from taking pramlintide up to 3 to 7 days, the doctor may increase its dose from time to time to obtain effective control of blood sugar.

Point to remember: pramlintide does not replace insulin; it is added to mealtime insulin to achieve better control of blood sugar in diabetes.

7

Treating Type 2 Diabetes with Pills

Treatment of diabetes with oral drugs or pills has certain features:

- Diabetes pills do not lower blood sugar in type 1 diabetes. They help control blood sugar in type 2 diabetes. For safety reasons, diabetes pills are not used during pregnancy.
- When lifestyle modification, including diet, weight loss, and exercise together fail to control blood sugar in type 2 diabetes, treatment with diabetes pills may be started.
- Most diabetes pills may be used alone (monotherapy) or combined with diabetes pills from other classes. In combination, the pills from different classes have an additive effect in lowering blood sugar.
- Treatment of a person with the newly diagnosed type 2 diabetes usually starts with a single medicine from the sulfonylurea class. If one kind of pill under the sulfonylurea class does not lower blood sugar; change it, and try another kind of pill from the sulfonylurea class.
- If sulfonylurea drugs alone fail to control blood sugar, successive combinations of diabetes pills from other classes may be tried.
- In selection of diabetes pills, factors such as the risk of low blood sugar, contraindication, and side effects should be considered.

- During treatment with diabetes pills, self-monitoring of blood sugar, hemoglobin A1C testing, and periodic monitoring of liver function are generally recommended.
- Long use of diabetes pills may decrease their effect, and a stage may come when the pills are not effective in controlling blood sugar. In this condition, your doctor may advise you to add insulin injection to the pills.
- Over time, type 2 diabetes exhausts beta cells of the pancreas, and as a result, the cells stop producing insulin. In the absence of natural insulin in the body, diabetes pills are ineffective in controlling blood sugar. At this stage, the pills should be discontinued and full-fledged insulin therapy must be started. Medical treatment of type 2 diabetes is gradually intensified to achieve good control of blood sugar (see table).

Diabetes pills are an aid and not a replacement for healthy eating and exercise in treatment of type 2 diabetes. However, different kinds of diabetes pills available today have provided remarkable options for managing type 2 diabetes.

Medical Treatment of Type 2 Diabetes	
Stage 1	Lifestyle modification, diet, and exercise (No drug)
Stage 2	Lifestyle modification, diet, and exercise plus use of one oral drug: sulfonylurea or biguanide
Stage 3	Lifestyle modification, diet, and exercise plus drug combination (add a second drug): sulfonylurea + biguanide or sulfonylurea or biguanide + alpha-glucosidase inhibitor or sulfonylurea or biguanide + thiazolidine or exenatide (Byetta) or biguanide + repaglinide or nateglinide or biguanide or thiazolidine + sitagliptin
Stage 4	insulin with oral drug: biguanide + insulin or thiazolidinedione + insulin or sulfonylurea + insulin or biguanide + thiazolidinedione + insulin
Stage 5	insulin alone
Stage 6	insulin+pramlintide
Source: DoD. *Clinical Practice Guidelines.*2003. *Epocrates.* 2007.	

8

The Basics of Insulin Therapy

Treatment of diabetes with insulin is called insulin therapy. Insulin is injected or inhaled to control raised blood sugar. A good control of blood sugar, in turn, reduces the risk for organ damage from diabetes.

WHO NEEDS INSULIN TREATMENT

The people listed below must take insulin injections or inhaled insulin to control their blood sugar:

- All people with type 1 diabetes. These people must inject or inhale insulin to remain alive because the pancreas does not produce insulin in type 1 diabetes. If these people do not inject insulin, their blood sugar will become very high, leading to dangerously high levels of acids in the blood (ketoacidosis). Such a condition can cause blood poisoning, and even death.
- People with type 2 diabetes when:
  - Nutrition, exercise, and diabetes pills have failed to control their blood sugar.
  - They have experienced rapid loss of weight.
  - Ketones are persistently present in their urine in a non-fasting state.
- Pregnant women with diabetes. Diabetes pills, for safety concerns, are not used to control diabetes in pregnancy.

Insulin, when injected or inhaled, lowers blood sugar in two ways: it moves sugar from your blood and delivers it to the cells of your body; and prevents production of sugar by your liver. Both these actions lower blood sugar levels.

SOURCES OF MANUFACTURED INSULIN

The insulin used in injections is either animal insulin or the synthetic insulin called human insulin. Inhaled insulin is also a synthetic insulin. Human insulin is the most common form of insulin used today.

Animal Insulin

Insulin is extracted from the pancreases of slaughtered cows or pigs. This was the only source of obtaining insulin till 1978 when synthetic insulin was invented. Although animal insulin was generally well tolerated by people, it sometimes caused a skin rash and inflammation at the injection site, probably due to differences in the chemical structure of animal insulin and the natural insulin in the human body.

Human Insulin

Human insulin is not derived from human beings; it is a synthetic product chemically manufactured in laboratories through a chemical process called recombinant DNA technology. The synthetic insulin is called human insulin because its chemical structure is exactly the same as that of insulin produced by the human body. Human insulin is more rapid in action than animal insulin, but it has a shorter duration of action. Because human insulin is well tolerated, its use is preferred for pregnant women, people allergic to animal insulin, and those who are just starting the insulin treatment. The synthetically manufactured human insulin has now almost completely replaced the animal insulin.

TYPES OF INSULIN

Based on how quickly the insulin is absorbed into the bloodstream after injection, and how long it remains active, human insulin is divided into four main types: rapid-acting, short-acting, intermediate-acting, and long-acting. (Substances are added in insulin to slow down its action.) In addition to these four main types, insulin mixtures of intermediate-acting and short-acting (regular) insulin, and intermediate-acting and rapid-acting insulin are also available. The actual time any type of insulin will take to work or remain active may differ in various persons and in different situations.

As for inhaled insulin, it is a rapid-acting insulin quickly absorbed in the blood after inhaling. (Find more about inhaled insulin in title 9.1).

9

Insulin Charts

The following charts outline the key features of different types of insulin taken through injections. However, check with your doctor because the features may vary slightly.

Rapid-Acting Insulin	
Names:	*Insulin lispro (Humalog)* *Insulin aspart (Novolog)* *Insulin glulisine (Apidra)*
Appearance:	Clear
Begins to work:	Less than 30 minutes (lispro) Less than 15 minutes (aspart) Less than 30 minutes (glulisine)
Peak action:	30 to 90 minutes (lispro) 1 to 3 hours (aspart) 30 to 90 minutes (glulisine)
Maximum duration:	Less than 6 hours (lispro) 3 to 5 hours (aspart) Less than 6 hours (glulisine)
Comment:	Inject it about 15 minutes before a meal.

Short-Acting Insulin	
Names:	*Regular insulin (Humulin R, Novolin R, Actrapid)*
Appearance:	Clear
Begins to work:	30 to 60 minutes
Peak action:	2 to 4 hours
Maximum duration:	6 to 12 hours
Comment:	Inject it 30 to 60 minutes before a meal.

Intermediate-Acting Insulin	
Names:	*NPH insulin (Humulin N, Novolin N)*
Appearance:	Cloudy Letter N on the bottle
Begins to work:	1 to 2 hours
Peak action:	4 to 14 hours
Maximum duration:	10 to less than 24 hours
Comment:	Inject it 30 to 60 minutes before a meal. This insulin may be combined with rapid-acting or short-acting insulin.
Lente and ultralente insulins have been discontinued.	

Long-Acting Insulin	
Names:	*Insulin glargine (Lantus)* *Insulin detemir (Levemir)*
Appearance:	Clear
Begins to work:	1 hour
Peak action:	No peak time
Maximum duration:	24 hours (glargine) 6 to 23 hours (detemir): dose dependent duration
Comment:	Do not mix it with any other type of insulin in the same syringe.
Source: Adapted from *Epocrates*, 2007.	

Insulin Mixtures	
70% NPH / 30% Regular :	(Humulin 70/30, Novolin 70/30)
50% NPH / 50% Regular :	Humulin 50/50
75% insulin lispro protamine/ 25% insulin lispro : (It is a mixture of intermediate-acting insulin lispro protamine and rapid-acting insulin lispro.)	(Humalog 75/25)

more...

<table>
<tr><td>70% insulin aspart protamine/
30% insulin aspart:
(It is a mixture of intermediate-acting insulin aspart protamine and rapid-acting insulin aspart.)</td><td>Novolog 70/30</td></tr>
<tr><td>50% insulin lispro protamine/
50% insulin lispro:</td><td>Humalog 50/50</td></tr>
<tr><td colspan="2">Comment:
• All these insulins are cloudy; do not mix them with any any other insulin.
• If the insulin mixture includes regular insulin, inject it 30 to 45 minutes before a meal; if the mixture contains rapid-acting insulin, inject it 15 minutes before your meal</td></tr>
</table>

9.1

Inhaled Insulin

Exubera is a rapid-acting dry insulin powder, which you inhale (breathe in through your mouth) using an inhaler. The inhaler is supplied with the inhaled insulin. Exubera is a human (synthetic) insulin that helps control blood sugar in adults with type 1 and type 2 diabetes.

How It Works

When you inhale insulin, it directly goes into your lungs from where it enters the bloodstream. Inhaled insulin enters the blood more rapidly than insulin injected under the skin. Inhaled insulin, like your own natural insulin, controls blood sugar.

Important Facts

- Exubera should be inhaled within 10 minutes before eating a meal.
- Inhaled insulin begins to work in about 10 to 20 minutes after inhalation; its action peaks in 2 hours; and its duration lasts for about 6 hours.
- Exubera when used by itself for 12 weeks has been shown to reduce A1C levels (the average amount of your blood sugar during the last 2 to 3 months) by about 2.2 percent.
- Inhaled insulin is only one part of a broad treatment plan

for diabetes. The other parts of the plan include healthy diet, regular exercise, and frequent checking of blood sugar.

- To control blood sugar, people with type 2 diabetes may take Exubera as a single medicine, or combine it with diabetes pills, or take some longer-acting insulin such as glargine or detemir in addition to Exubera. People with type 1 diabetes will need to take a longer-acting insulin in addition to Exubera.

Risk for low blood sugar

As with other forms of insulin, Exubera may lead to low blood sugar.

Effect on blood fats

Triglycerides decrease in people taking Exubera.

Main Side Effect

Cough. Exubera may also lower your lung function.

Other possible side effects

These include chest pain (unrelated to heart disease), dry mouth, and ear pain.

Dose

Start inhaled insulin with 0.05 mg per 1 kg of body weight, three times a day, before each meal.

Exubera comes in single dose blister packs of 1 mg or 3 mg of insulin, which you insert in the inhaler supplied with the medicine. When you pierce the blister, insulin powder scatters into the chamber of the inhaler and is ready for inhaling.

Caution

Below listed people should not use Exubera:

- Children and teenagers. Exubera has not been tested in these people.
- Smokers or those who quit smoking less than 6 months ago.
- People with lung problems such as asthma.
- Women who are pregnant or plan to be pregnant. Exubera may be harmful to the unborn baby. Check with the doctor before taking inhaled insulin in pregnancy.

Because Exubera may make your lung function weak, the doctor will advise you to have a lung function test before starting Exubera, and from time to time while staying with its treatment.

IMPORTANT. Exubera could not become popular among customers and physicians because of several downsides of the product: risk of lung cancer, use of an awkward big inhaler, high cost, and the development of alternative agents of controlling blood sugar. As a result, Pfizer, the manufacturing company of Exubera, has stopped production of this drug. Exubera will no longer be available as of September 1, 2008.

10

Elements of Insulin Therapy

Here are the key elements of insulin therapy administered through insulin injections:

Mixing of insulins

Use of mixed insulins may be more effective in regulating blood sugar than injecting insulin of a single type. Many people take a combination of short-acting and long-acting insulins at the same time in one injection.

Today, "premixed" insulins of several types are available. However, if you self-mix insulins, first draw the short-acting insulin in the syringe; then draw in the required amount of the long-acting insulin from the other bottle. By mixing insulin in this order, transparency of the short-acting insulin will not be soiled with the clouded particles present in the long-acting insulin. If you reverse this order, and draw in the long-acting insulin first and then enter the syringe needle in the bottle of the short-acting insulin, the cloudy particles of the long-acting insulin will slow down the effect of the short-acting insulin.

Standard guidelines on mixing of insulins and the use of these mixtures are:

- Generally, short-acting (regular) insulin should not be mixed with the long-acting insulins. Substances in the long-acting insulins slow down the onset of the short-acting insulin.

- Intermediate-acting insulin (NPH) may be mixed with the short-acting (regular) insulin.
- Rapid-acting insulin can be mixed with either the intermediate-acting or the long-acting insulin.
- Mixing of rapid-acting insulin with the long-acting insulin does not reduce the onset of the rapid-acting insulin.
- Do not mix long-acting insulin glargine or insulin detemir with any other type of insulin because it may alter the insulin action.
- Do not mix buffered insulin with any other insulin because the buffering ingredient may affect the insulin activity.
- When your blood sugar is well controlled on a particular mixture of insulin, continue with that mixture.
- You may use premixed commercial insulin if the combination is according to your insulin requirement.

Injection Sites

Insulin is injected in the fatty tissue under the skin (subcutaneous tissue). Injecting insulin through the muscle or vein is not recommended for daily use. Injecting insulin through these routes is not only inconvenient in self-administration, but may also accelerate insulin action so fast that blood sugar may fall too low. These methods are generally used in emergency conditions in a hospital to bring down extremely high blood sugar levels such as in ketoacidosis. In insulin-injection therapy:

- Insulin can be injected in the upper arm, thigh, buttock, or the abdomen around 2 inches away from the navel. How fast insulin is absorbed in your body depends upon the site where it is injected. Insulin is absorbed fastest at the abdomen, then arms, thighs, and slowest at the buttocks. Exercise enhances the absorption rate of the injected insulin by increasing blood flow at the injection sties. If you inject insulin in your arm, for example, exercising the arm will cause insulin to work quickly.

- Rotate injection sites. Injecting insulin repeatedly at the same spot makes the skin tissue hard, and slow down the absorption rate of the injected insulin. If you inject in the abdomen, for example, rotate around the different spots on the abdomen.

Insulin Units

Insulin dosage is expressed in units (U).

Insulin Strength

In the United States, insulin is currently available in the strengths of U-100 and U-500. These strengths express the number of insulin units in 1 milliliter (1cc) of solution. The insulin of U-100 is the most common; one insulin bottle contains 10 milliliters (ml) of liquid insulin, that is, a total of 1,000 units in a bottle. Insulin strength of U-500 is very strong; it is used in extreme conditions only when regular strength insulin is ineffective and fails to reduce high blood sugar.

Insulin Storage

Insulin bottles and cartridges (used in insulin pens) should be stored properly. Follow storage instructions that come with your insulin bottle or cartridge. Generally:

- Unopened insulin bottles and cartridges should be kept in a refrigerator, not a freezer.
- In-use insulin bottles and cartridges can be used up to 3 months when stored in a refrigerator, and up to 1 month

when kept at room temperatures below 86°F (30°C) and protected from sunlight. Insulin should not be kept at extreme temperatures.

- Insulin potency is reduced if an opened insulin bottle is kept at room temperature for more than 1 month. If you use insulin of reduced potency, blood sugar will not be properly controlled.
- Insulin should not be used after its expiration date. If insulin in the bottle decomposes even before the expiration date (clear insulin becomes frosty and frosty becomes clumpy), discard the insulin bottle.

Insulin and X-Ray Security

Normally, when your insulin bottles are passed through X-ray machines at airports, the insulin remains unaffected. But, if the bottle remains exposed to these rays for a longer time or is exposed repeatedly to the X-rays, stability of the insulin can be affected.

Insulin Delivery

The most common methods of insulin delivery include the traditional syringe and needle system, insulin pens, and insulin pump (more about these methods in the following titles).

11

Methods of Insulin Delivery

Today, the methods for administering insulin are:

- Syringe and needle system
- Insulin pen
- Insulin injector
- Insulin pump
- Inhaled insulin

SYRINGE AND NEEDLE SYSTEM

The syringe and needle is the most common form of insulin delivery. (In the United States, the system of disposable syringe with pre-attached needle is very common.) Some features of this system are:

- Insulin syringes are available in various sizes, including 2cc (200 units), 1cc (100 units), 1/2 cc (50 units), 1/3 cc (30 units), and 1/4 cc (25 units).
- The smallest syringe that can hold your insulin dose can make it easier for you to draw in your accurate dose.
- Syringe needles are available in several lengths. Changes in the needle length may alter insulin absorption in your body.

- Glass syringes and needles should be sterilized every time they are reused.
- Disposable syringes are designated for one time use. The American Diabetes Association (ADA), however, holds that reuse of these syringes is safe if done under proper hygienic conditions. For safe reuse, flush the syringe with air 2 to 3 times to remove any insulin sticking on its walls or the needle. Do not wipe the needle with alcohol, because doing so may impair its protective coating. Recap the needle and store the syringe at normal room temperature for the next use. Present day disposable syringes contain thinner needles and are meant to be used once only. People at increased risk of getting infections should not reuse a syringe or an insulin pen needle. Do not reuse a needle that has become blunt.
- Used syringes and needles must be disposed of properly by placing and sealing them in a safe container before throwing them in trash cans. Several needle cutting devices are available that you can use to cut and store syringe and pen needles for later disposal.

INSULIN PEN

An insulin pen is like a pen, containing inside a cartridge of insulin, and a fine needle at its top. Some pens use replaceable cartridges while others are totally disposable. Insulin pens are becoming increasingly popular (more in title 11.2).

INSULIN JET INJECTOR

An insulin jet injector does not use needles. This device sends a fine spray or mist of insulin beneath the skin by a high-pressure air mechanism instead of needles. The spray pressure used in these devices may cause pain or bruising at the injection site, especially in thin people. The insulin injectors have to be sterilized usually every week.

INSULIN PUMP

The insulin pump is worn on the body (not implanted inside the body). The pump delivers insulin in the body continuously, day and night (more in title 11.3).

INHALED INSULIN

Inhaled insulin has already been discussed in title 9.1.

Experiments to perfect other convenient ways of insulin delivery without injections such as an insulin pill and insulin skin patches are under active development. Insulin pills have been developed, which, unaffected by the stomach enzymes, will be absorbed into the bloodstream. Insulin through skin patches will be directly absorbed into the blood through the skin. The results of these experiments are encouraging. These convenient and noninvasive ways of insulin delivery, if perfected, will make diabetes management easy and less painful.

11.1

Insulin Self-Injecting Technique

Most people use syringes to self-inject insulin under the skin. When you use the regular syringe-and-needle system, two steps are taken to self-inject insulin: first, you prepare the insulin dose, and then you inject this dose.

PREPARING THE INSULIN DOSE

To prepare the injection, wash your hands with soap and water. Inspect the insulin bottle to make sure that insulin inside the bottle is not decomposed. (Clear insulin becomes frosty and frosty becomes lumpy when decomposed. Such changes cause loss of insulin potency.) Prepare the insulin injection as shown in the following figures.

1. Roll the insulin bottle (except rapid-acting and short-acting insulins) between the palms of your hands to mix the contents. Do not shake the bottle because shaking can decompose the contents.

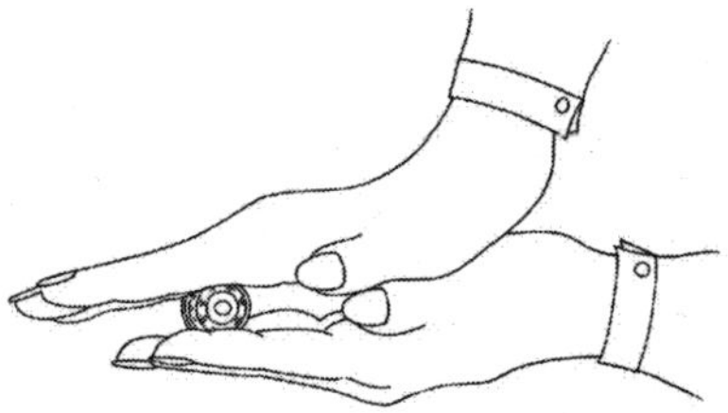

1

2. Clean the rubber top of the insulin bottle with an alcohol swab, and let the top dry.

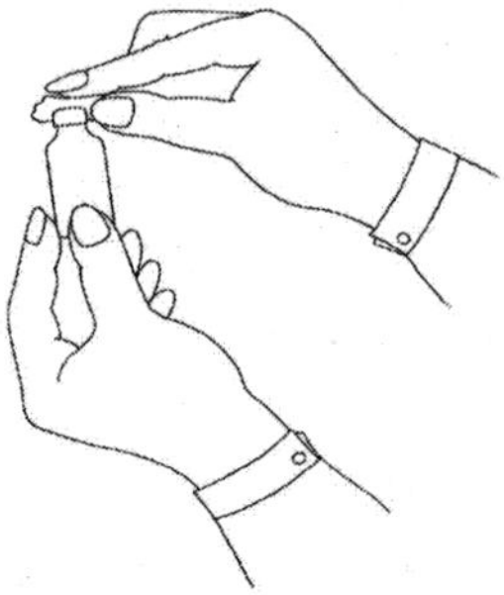

2

3. Draw air in the syringe by pulling the syringe plunger back until the top edge of the plunger aligns at the level or the number of units matching your dose.

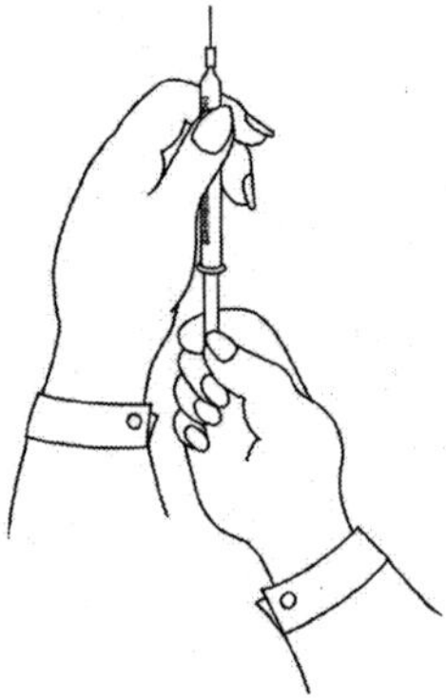

3

4. Inject the needle into the rubber top of the insulin bottle, push the plunger down letting the air go into the bottle.

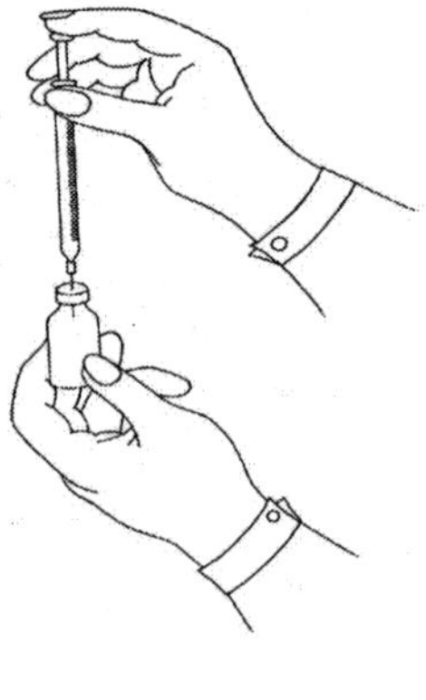

4

5. Turn the bottle upside down resting on the top of the needle; the tip of the needle will be inside the contents of the bottle. Holding the bottle with one hand, pull the plunger back with the other, drawing in the correct dose of insulin into the syringe. Before removing the syringe from the bottle, check your syringe for air bubbles (bubbles reduce the amount of insulin). If air bubbles are present, tap the side of the syringe with your finger and let the bubbles go out of the needle in the bottle. Withdraw the correct dose. Take out the needle from the bottle; lay the syringe down in a manner that the needle does not touch anything. You are now ready to take the insulin injection.

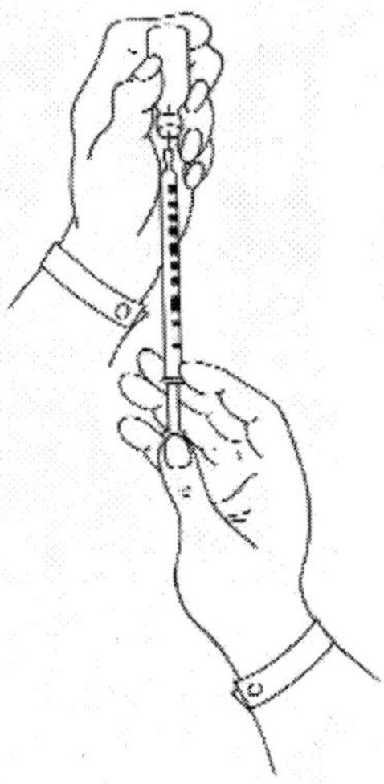

5

TAKING THE INJECTION

To self-inject insulin:

- Select the site on your body where you will inject insulin. This site can be the upper arms, abdomen, thighs or buttocks. The sites on the front of the body where you can easily self-inject are shown in the figure below. (The actual point where you inject should be changed with each injection.)
- Clean the skin at the chosen site with alcohol. Before you inject, let the skin be dry.

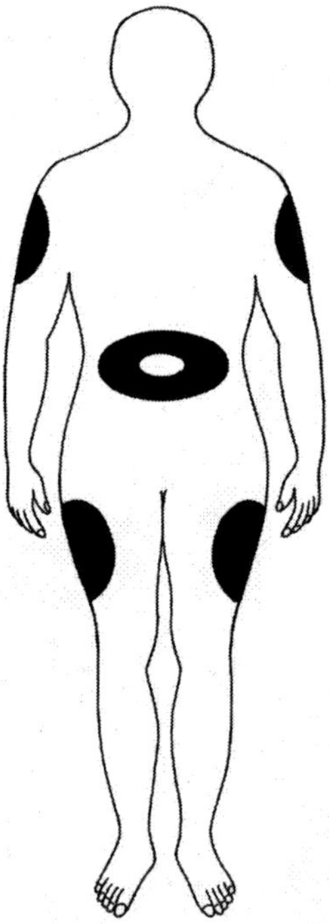

Sites (marked) for self-injecting insulin

- Grip the skin fold between your fingers of one hand; holding the syringe in the other hand like a pencil, insert the needle straightaway into the gripped skin.
- Push down the plunger slowly, releasing insulin inside the body till the full dose is injected.
- Release the gripped skin; hold the needle inside the skin for a few seconds to make sure that all the insulin is injected, and then pull out the needle straightaway.
- Press the injection site with a cotton swab for a few seconds to reduce bleeding if any; do not rub the skin.
- If a blood drop comes out after taking out the needle, press the site with a dry cotton for several seconds.

PREPARING AN INJECTION WITH MIXED INSULINS

Unless you are using "premixed insulin," you can prepare a mixture of short-acting and long-acting insulins for your injection as follows:

- Wash your hands with soap and water.
- Clean the rubber tops of both insulin bottles with an alcohol swab; let the tops of the bottles dry.
- Draw air into the syringe equal to the units of long-acting insulin you will take. Inject the air into the long-acting insulin bottle. Do not draw insulin in the syringe. Take out the needle from the bottle.
- Next, draw air into the syringe equal to the units of short-acting insulin you will take. Inject the air into the short-acting insulin bottle. Turn the bottle upside down, resting on the top of the needle; the tip of the needle will be inside the contents of the bottle.

- Holding the bottle with one hand, pull the plunger back with the other, drawing your correct dose of short-acting insulin in the syringe. Remove any air bubbles by tapping the syringe with your finger, and let the bubbles go out of the needle into the bottle.
- Remove the needle from the bottle and lay the syringe without touching any surface.
- Next, roll the long-acting insulin bottle between the palms of your hands so that the contents are mixed.
- Insert the needle into the long-acting insulin bottle. Turn the bottle upside down resting on the top of the needle; the tip of the needle will be inside the bottle's contents.
- Holding the bottle with one hand, pull the plunger back with the other, drawing in the long-acting insulin to the extent that insulin in your syringe equals the total dose of short-acting and long acting insulins. (If you draw in a dose of long-acting insulin greater than your need, do not push it back into the bottle; throw it away, and prepare the dose again with an empty syringe.) Take out the needle from the long-acting insulin bottle.
- You are now ready to take the insulin injection.
- To inject, follow the steps of injecting insulin noted before.

HOW TO MINIMIZE INJECTION PAIN

Here are some helpful tips:

- Do not inject cold insulin. Keep the insulin bottle at room temperature before injecting.
- Do not use cold or hot needles.
- Before injecting, make sure the syringe has no bubbles.

- Be relaxed, do not tense muscles in the injecting site.
- Insert the needle quickly in the skin.
- Do not reuse blunt needles.
- Do not inject insulin in the areas usually red or itchy.

CAUTION

- Because insulin therapy may cause low blood sugar, always carry with you some kind of quick-acting carbohydrate such as glucose tablets for immediate treatment of falling blood sugar.
- Also, carry with you some kind of identification: keep a card in your pocket, or wear a bracelet or necklace stating that you have diabetes. This can assist other people in providing you treatment in an emergency situation when your blood sugar falls too low and you are unable to treat yourself.

11.2

Insulin Pen

An insulin pen, about the size of a large marker, is a device for injecting insulin (see fig. on the following page). The pen contains insulin in a self-contained cartridge, and a fine needle placed at its top. The needle is usually kept separate from the pen and is attached only at the time of injection.The insulin pens are of two main types— reusable and disposable. In a reusable pen, you reuse the pen portion but replace a new cartridge when insulin has been used. Such a pen can last for several years. As for a disposable pen, you throw it away when its prefilled insulin cartridge becomes empty. Insulin pens are available for many types of insulin such as:

- Rapid-acting (aspart, lispro, and glulisine)
- Regular short-acting
- Long-acting (glargine and glulisine)
- Certain insulin mixtures —70/30, 75/25, and 50/50

The pens are available in many brands and models. Check with your doctor which pen will be right for you.

Important Notes:

- Pens are available for many types of insulin. Check if pens are available for the insulin you are taking.

Disposable Insulin Pen

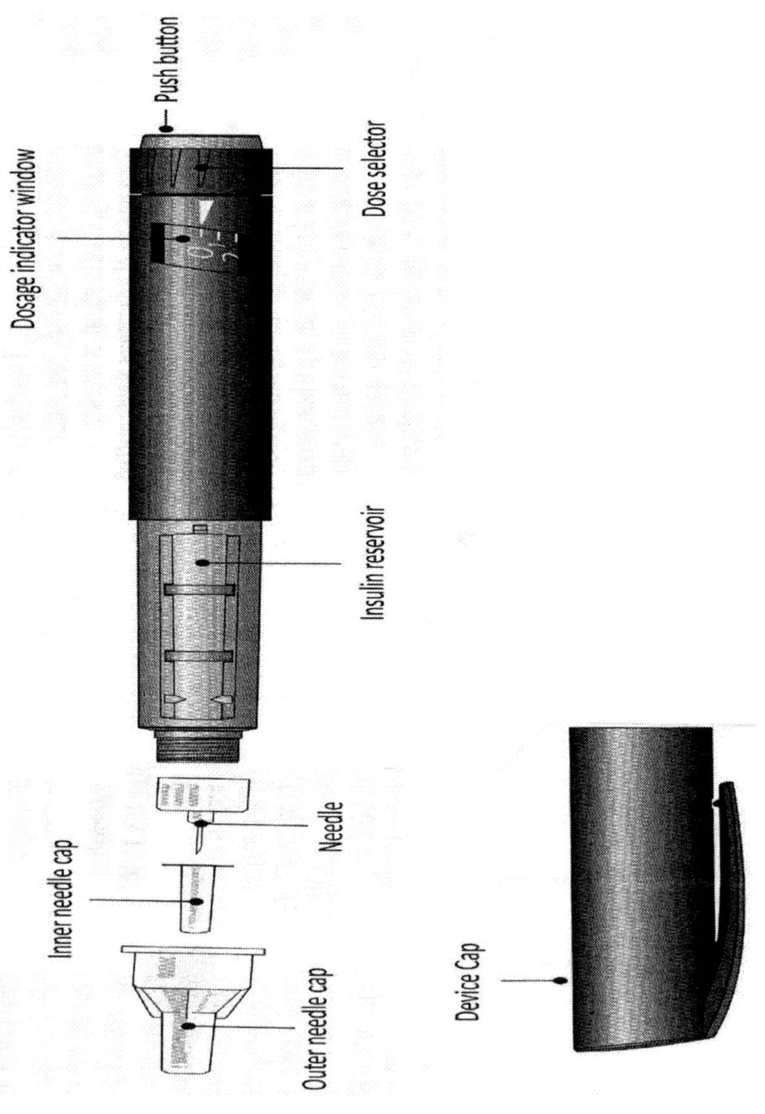

- An insulin pen takes little preparation time. While using the pen, you do not need to fill insulin in the syringe, it comes prefilled in a cartridge.
- The pens are easy to carry, require a few or no extra supplies, and are desirable for people who want to take insulin injection in an easy, fast, and private way.
- Insulin pens are easy to operate. You turn the dial to select the desired dose of insulin, place the pen needle into the skin, and using thumb pressure, push in the injector button to deliver the insulin. And you are done.
- The insulin pens usually deliver accurate doses.
- Each time you use the pen to inject insulin, attach a new needle on the pen. However, some people choose to use a needle for more than once.
- The pen in use should be kept at room temperature, away from bright light. Do not keep it in a refrigerator.
- Prefilled Insulin pens and insulin cartridges— not in use— should be kept in a refrigerator (not in a freezer) until the expiration date.
- Storing the pen with needle attached may cause air and bubble enter the insulin cartridge. The extra air and bubble may lead to injecting wrong amount of insulin.
- A disposable insulin pen is generally more convenient than a reusable pen because you do not need to load a new cartridge.
- Insulin pen system is more expensive than the syringe bottle system.
- Insulin cartridges used in the United States hold 150 or 300 units of insulin. Most disposable pens contain 300 units of insulin.

- To prevent infection, do not share your insulin pen with other users.

The insulin pens come with "step-by-step instructions" on how to use them for injecting insulin.

11.3

The Insulin Pump

The aim of insulin therapy is to provide the body with insulin that is lacking in diabetes. Sometimes, however, even three or more insulin injections taken per day may fail to control blood sugar. In such a situation, an insulin pump that continuously delivers insulin in the body may be considered to replace multiple insulin injections. The insulin pump aims to mimic a healthy pancreas in its insulin delivery.

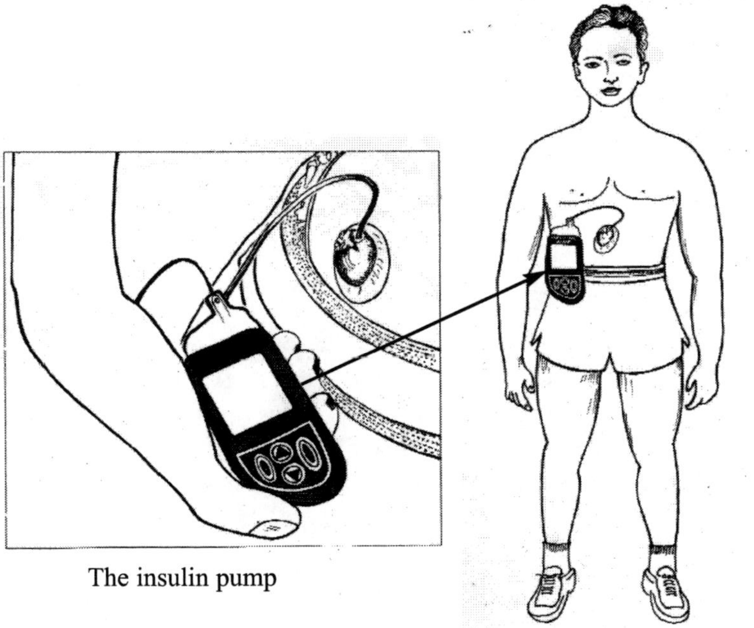

The insulin pump

PUMP DESCRIPTION

The insulin pump, which is about the size of a beeper, is a battery-powered device of insulin delivery. The user wears the pump on the body in a pouch or on a belt holder all the time, round the clock. The pump consists of a reservoir (syringe) filled with insulin, a small battery-operated pump, and a computer chip that allows the user to regulate how much insulin the pump should deliver. A plastic case contains all these components. A thin plastic tube called an infusion set is attached to the pump, and on the other end of the tube a needle or soft catheter called cannula is attached. The cannula is inserted under the skin, usually on the abdomen, to deliver insulin continuously in the body. The infusion set is kept at a site for 2 to 3 days and then moved to a new site.

Although the pump is to be used throughout day and night, you may manage to keep it off for 1 to 2 hours such as when going for swimming or performing a sexual activity. But take an injection of regular insulin to cover your insulin requirement during the period when you are off the pump. Your healthcare professional will help you learn how to program the pump for delivering insulin at regular intervals.

INSULIN DELIVERY THROUGH INSULIN PUMP

Because the insulin pump continuously delivers insulin in the body through the skin, this kind of insulin delivery is also called continuous subcutaneous insulin infusion (CSII). The word "subcutaneous" refers to "beneath the skin." The insulin pump, however, is not automatic; you have to program it for how much insulin it has to deliver. The pump uses only rapid-acting or short-acting insulin; it does not use long-acting or mixed insulins. The pump delivers insulin in two different modes: basal and bolus modes.

Basal Delivery

The insulin pump delivers tiny amounts of insulin continuously, day and night, approximately in the same way as the pancreas of a normal healthy person does. This is called basal delivery. You can program the pump to deliver insulin at various basal rates at different times of the day. For example, when your requirement of insulin decreases such as during an exercise, you may reduce the basal rate. Again, when you are under stress, your insulin requirement may increase, and you may increase the basal rate. How much basal rate is right for you? Your healthcare professional will determine the right dose for you after assessing your specific requirement for insulin. Some people may need a basal rate as low as 0.5 unit per hour.

In newer insulin pumps, you can adjust the basal rates very precisely in as little as 0.05 unit per hour. Such adjustments are ideal for those people whose daily need of insulin is limited. Nearly 40 to 50 percent of your total daily dose of insulin may be used in basal delivery; the remaining 50 to 60 percent of the insulin dose is delivered in divided doses before the breakfast, lunch, and dinner.

Bolus Delivery

Bolus is a large dose of insulin. When you take meals or snacks, your body needs more insulin to process the food than what the pump secretes in tiny amounts in the basal mode. In insulin pump therapy, you will deliver the bolus dose through your pump. (The pump will not do it automatically.) What should be the amount of the bolus dose? This decision is made by you, not by the insulin pump. Assume that you have learned from your experience that 1 unit of short-acting insulin covers 15 grams of carbohydrate (such as 1 slice of bread) in your diet. This means that to cover an intake of 90 grams of carbohydrate, you will program your pump to deliver a bolus of 6 units of insulin.

PRESENT DAY INSULIN PUMPS

Insulin pump technology has greatly improved during the last 40 years. (Insulin pumps came in the 1960s.) The newer pumps have become smaller in size and are more precise than before. These pumps contain pre-filled insulin cartridges, have remote programmers attached for injecting large doses of insulin when required (bolusing), and can transmit data of several weeks to a computer for analysis. A device that combines a glucose meter and an insulin pump with a dose calculator is also available. When using this device, you put a blood drop on a test strip and insert it into a monitor from where the blood sugar level is sent by a wireless signal to the insulin pump. The dose calculator in the pump then recommends an insulin dose on the basis of your blood sugar reading. Then, you simply push a button on your pump to deliver the calculated dose.

IMPLANTABLE INSULIN PUMP

An insulin pump has been developed, which is implanted inside the body. A tiny sensor in this pump detects when blood sugar is rising in the body, and instructs the pump to release insulin directly into the abdomen from where it is quickly absorbed. Scientists in the United States are using this pump for research purposes.

11.4

Insulin Pump Again

As a device of insulin delivery, the insulin pump offers several advantages, including:

Tight Control of Blood Sugar

The insulin pump delivers small amounts of insulin continuously round-the-clock and injects larger doses when you require an additional amount of insulin such as to cover a meal. The pump can be programmed to deliver low doses of insulin during the night to prevent low blood sugar, and increase the doses toward the morning to keep blood sugar in check in the fasting state.

Insulin pump therapy can be especially beneficial in pregnancy because it helps achieve tight control of blood sugar. A good control of blood sugar in pregnancy leads to preventing pregnancy complications from diabetes and helps achieve normal deliveries.

Convenience

Intensive insulin therapy through insulin pump is more convenient than the intensive therapy through multiple insulin injections. In multiple injection treatment, you inject insulin several times a day to control blood sugar. This is an inconvenient task. The insulin pump solves this inconvenience because insulin is injected only once in the pump's reservoir that is sufficient for 2 to 3 days.

Flexibility

The insulin pump, by delivering large and small doses of insulin, allows you to have a flexible lifestyle. Before you eat a meal, you press buttons on the pump to deliver a large dose (bolus) of short-acting insulin for covering peaks of blood sugar after eating. However, when you miss a meal, you do not deliver a large dose, and the pump continues releasing small doses of insulin (basal delivery). The continuous delivery of insulin in small doses is so tiny that it does not cause low blood sugar even if you miss a meal. This feature of flexibility of insulin administration in the insulin pump is missing in the insulin injections.

WHO NEEDS THE INSULIN PUMP

The insulin pump is not for every diabetic person. However, it may be beneficial for those people with diabetes:

- Whose blood sugar is not controlled despite multiple insulin injections.
- Who either have low blood sugar during the night or raised blood sugar in the morning.
- Who are highly motivated to keep a tight control of their blood sugar, and are ready to take extra care for proper maintenance of their insulin pumps.
- Who are willing to self-test their blood sugar frequently (at least four times a day) to monitor control of their blood sugar while using the insulin pump.
- Who know that the function of the insulin pump is just to deliver insulin as they program it, and that they themselves have to take care of their diet, exercise, and medication to control blood sugar.
- Who, because of their variable work schedules, cannot plan their meals and determine timings of their meals

and insulin injections. Insulin pumps provide the flexibility of insulin delivery.

- Who, when pregnant, aim for tight control of their blood sugar to achieve safe pregnancies.

LIMITATIONS OF THE PUMP

These include:

- The insulin pump by itself cannot measure blood sugar, nor can it automatically change the dose of insulin to control blood sugar. Pump users have to self-monitor their blood sugar frequently. Based on the results of this monitoring, they adjust the amount of insulin they should take by regulating the settings of their pumps.
- The pump may malfunction for some technical problem without your ever knowing it. Some time back, Disetronic Medical Systems issued a recall of all of their D-TRON insulin pumps because a problem had developed in their insulin delivery mechanism.
- The insulin pump may clog and fail to work. When the pump stops working, it will not release insulin, leading to uncontrolled peaks of blood sugar. As a result, acids may become too high in the blood, causing diabetic ketoacidosis (DKA), a serious medical emergency in diabetes. Present day insulin pumps, however, have added features that signal technical problems, which you can correct by taking timely action.
- Pump users have to be extra careful in personal hygiene. Because the infusion set continuously remains at one site of the body for 2 to 3 days, swelling and infection may occur at the site of infusion. However, careful hygiene, rotation of infusion sites, and timely use of antibiotics help resolve such problems.

- One argument that questions the use of insulin pumps is that blood sugar control achieved by the pump can probably be obtained by conventional injection therapy. For example, injecting the long-acting insulin glargine or insulin detemir for your basal insulin need, and taking the rapid-acting insulin lispro, aspart, or glulisine before each meal may have the same effect as provided by the basal and bolus deliveries of the insulin pump.
- For some people, wearing the insulin pump continuously and incorporating it into the daily life may be a challenging task.

Most people, changing from conventional insulin injections to using insulin pumps, achieve better control of blood sugar, and reduce their risks for diabetes complications. Your doctor will determine if you need an insulin pump to control your blood sugar. If you are placed on the insulin pump therapy, you will require continued support from your healthcare professionals, at least in the beginning phase of the therapy. When you are using the insulin pump, keep the insulin syringes handy. You might need to resume injecting insulin under the skin, at least for a while, just in case the pump develops some problem. A healthcare professional or a diabetes educator will help you learn how to operate and use the insulin pump in treating diabetes.

12

Implementing Insulin Therapy

Insulin therapy or insulin regimen is based on planned use of insulin. The information presented here is about the most common method of insulin therapy — insulin injections. For inhaled insulin and the continuous infusion of insulin through an insulin pump, see titles 9.1 and 11.3. The key parts of insulin therapy are:

- Use of insulin injections
- Type of insulin to be used
- Dose or units of insulin to be injected
- Number of injections per day
- Timing of injections
- Self-monitoring of blood sugar

HOW MUCH INJECTABLE INSULIN DO YOU NEED

In diabetes, every person's requirement for insulin may be different, and it has to be individualized. The insulin need of people with type 2 diabetes will be different from people with type 1 diabetes, at least in the beginning. Your doctor will determine your daily insulin requirement, which in turn will depend on various factors, including the type of diabetes you have, your weight, your lifestyle, and the recent trends of your blood sugar.

The following treatment standards, however, are generally acceptable in the current medical practice:

- People with type 1 diabetes may take 0.5 unit of insulin per 1 kg of their body weight. By this formula, if you weigh 90 kgs, your total daily dose of insulin will amount to 45 units.
- For people with type 2 diabetes whose weight is in the BMI range of less than 27, the starting total daily dose of insulin may be 15 units.
- For people with a BMI of 27 or greater, the starting total daily dose of insulin may be 30 units.
- As type 2 diabetes becomes chronic, the insulin producing capacity of the pancreas gradually declines and a stage may come when an absolute deficiency of insulin can occur. In such a situation, the insulin requirement of people with type 2 diabetes will almost be the same as that of people with type 1 diabetes (more on this later).

DISTRIBUTING YOUR TOTAL DAILY INSULIN DOSE

Your doctor will advise you how to distribute your total daily dose of insulin in multiple injections that will be most suitable for you in controlling blood sugar. There can be several options, including:

Two-injection plan:

- Two-thirds of the total daily dose of insulin may be injected before breakfast.
- The remaining one-third may be injected before dinner.

- Each dose in this plan will consist of two parts of NPH and one part of regular insulin.

Three-injection plan:

- Two-thirds of the total daily dose of insulin may be injected before breakfast with two parts of NPH and one part of regular insulin.
- One-sixth of the total daily dose, comprising of regular insulin, may be injected before the evening meal.
- The remaining one-sixth of the total daily dose, comprising of NPH, may be injected before bedtime.

Flexible insulin plans:

- One-third of the total daily dose of insulin may be taken as NPH before bedtime. The remaining dose may be taken as regular insulin in divided doses before breakfast, lunch, and dinner; adjust the doses according to your blood sugar readings, changes in meals, exercise, and the amount of carbohydrate you will eat.

or

- Half of the total daily dose of insulin may be taken as background insulin (insulin glargine or insulin detemir) before breakfast or before bedtime. The remaining half may be taken in divided doses as insulin lispro, aspart, glulisine, or regular insulin before breakfast, lunch, and dinner. The insulin dose before each meal will depend on your blood sugar readings before meals and the amount of carbohydrate you will eat.

INSULIN-TO-CARBOHYDRATE RATIO

No formula exists that can exactly determine how many points of blood sugar will decline with 1 unit of insulin. You may, however, find from your experience that 1 unit of short-acting insulin covers 10 to 15 grams of carbohydrate. (Carbohydrate foods, as you know, are the main nutrients responsible for raising blood sugar.) Building on this experience, you will match the amount of your insulin dose with the amount of carbohydrate in your meals. Such a matching will help control your blood sugar and keep it within your target range. When you eat extra carbohydrate, your standard dose of insulin, however, will not be able to cover the resulting rise of blood sugar. In such a situation, a rule of thumb, known as the 1500-rule (see below), may be applied. This rule will help you determine how many points of blood sugar (resulting from eating extra amount of carbohydrates) will decline with each additional unit of regular insulin over and above your standard dose. To apply the 1500-rule:

- Get a total of how many units of all kinds of insulin (rapid-acting, short-acting, long-acting, and others) you inject per day. This is your total daily dose of insulin (TDD) that keeps your blood sugar under control. Assume the total is 30 units of insulin.

- Divide 1500 by 30. The result is 50, that is, 1 unit of short-acting insulin when added to your usual insulin dose will decrease 50 points of blood sugar.

Keep in mind, however, that the 1500-rule is a mere estimate of your insulin requirement and may differ from person to person and be different in varying situations.

ADJUSTING INSULIN THERAPY

If your blood sugar is high/low, the following adjustments in your insulin injections can be helpful:

- If your morning fasting blood sugar is high/low, increase/decrease the evening NPH.
- If your evening blood sugar is high/low, increase/decrease the morning NPH.
- If your evening glucose continues to be high/low, check your pre-lunch blood sugar.
- If your pre-lunch blood sugar is high/low, increase/ decrease the morning regular insulin.
- If your bedtime blood sugar is high/low, increase/decrease the evening regular insulin.

COMMON SIDE EFFECTS OF INSULIN THERAPY

These include:

- Low blood sugar. (This can be avoided by taking the right insulin in the right dose at the right time.)
- Weight gain. (This can be prevented by controlling your calorie intake and exercising regularly.)
- Swelling of the ankles, feet, and legs. This is a short-term side effect.)
- Redness, swelling, and itching at the site of injection. (These conditions usually clear up in a few days.)
- Thickening of tissues where you inject insulin. (Rotating the sites where you inject will help.)

12.1

Intensive Insulin Therapy

Intensive insulin therapy aims to keep a tight control on blood sugar. Well conducted studies have conclusively shown that by keeping blood sugar within the normal or near to normal range, people with type 1 and type 2 diabetes can prevent or at least delay the long-term complications of diabetes. You can use either insulin injections or an insulin pump in intensive insulin treatment. Intensive insulin therapy has certain features such as:

- You take multiple (three or more) insulin injections every day. In addition to short-acting or rapid-acting insulin, these injections consist of intermediate or long-acting insulin that provides background insulin.

or

- You wear a small insulin pump (discussed before) that continuously releases small amounts of short-acting or rapid-acting insulin in your body through a plastic tube. The pump allows you to give a large dose of insulin when you eat.

- Whether you take multiple insulin injections every day or use an insulin pump, self-monitor your blood sugar before each meal, and sometimes 2 to 3 hours after a meal. Blood sugar testing before meals guides you how much insulin you should inject to cover a meal. After-meal testing helps you learn how well your insulin therapy is controlling your blood sugar.

- Based on the results of your blood sugar testing, adjust your insulin dose, the amount of food you plan to eat, and the amount of exercise you expect to undertake.
- Intensive insulin therapy can have various combinations of insulin injections such as outlined in title 12.2.

INTENSIVE INSULIN THERAPY AND MEAL PLANNING

Intensive insulin therapy allows you to have a flexible meal plan in which you can adjust your insulin dose according to the carbohydrate content of your meals and snacks. If your meal is high in carbohydrates (which cause maximum rise of blood sugar), you will administer a greater dose of insulin to cover your meal. On the other hand, if you eat small amount of carbohydrates, you will inject a reduced dose of insulin. Or if you skip a meal, you will skip the insulin dose also. Note, however, if you take fixed doses of insulin every day, it is essential that you take meals containing the same amount of carbohydrate at about the same time daily for consistent control of your blood sugar.

LIMITATION OF INTENSIVE INSULIN THERAPY

Although intensive insulin therapy helps you control diabetes effectively, the therapy has limitations too. Intensive insulin therapy is not for every person who takes insulin injections to control blood sugar. If you are prone to low blood sugar, you may not be the right candidate for intensive insulin treatment. Such a therapy will further heighten your risk of low blood sugar. In addition, intensive insulin therapy cannot reverse or relieve a diabetes complication that has already reached its advanced stage (kidney failure, for example). Your doctor will evaluate if you are acandidate for intensive insulin treatment.

12.2

Insulin Therapy for Type 1 Diabetes

People with type 1 diabetes, as noted before, must take insulin because their bodies have stopped producing insulin. These people must get a well-designed and safe insulin treatment plan from their doctors. This is necessary because insulin therapy is associated with low blood sugar risk, and since these people must take insulin, they are at its excess risk.

There can be various options of insulin treatment, depending on the specific needs of the individuals. Some standard options of insulin treatment for people with type 1 diabetes are outlined on the following pages.

Insulin Plan 1			
Before Breakfast	*Before Lunch*	*Before Dinner*	*Before Bedtime*
Intermediate-acting NPH	–	Intermediate-acting NPH	–
This plan can be used by the newly diagnosed people with type 1 diabetes whose bodies are still producing some insulin. NPH taken in the morning provides background insulin during the day; when taken before dinner, it helps control fasting blood sugar the next morning.			

Insulin Plan 2			
Before Breakfast	*Before Lunch*	*Before Dinner*	*Before Bedtime*
Intermediate-acting NPH **plus** short-acting regular	–	Short-acting regular	Intermediate-acting NPH
Regular (short-acting) insulin before breakfast and dinner covers blood sugar after these meals. NPH in the morning provides basal or background insulin during the day. Bedtime NPH provides background insulin over night, and controls fasting blood sugar the next morning.			

Insulin Plan 3			
Before Breakfast	*Before Lunch*	*Before Dinner*	*Before Bedtime*
Intermediate-acting NPH **plus** rapid-acting lispro, aspart, or glulisine	Rapid-acting lispro, aspart, or glulisine	Rapid-acting lispro, aspart, or glulisine	Intermediate-acting NPH
This plan mimics the activity of a normal pancreas. It is an example of a flexible insulin regimen. This plan allows you to adjust the timing of your insulin injections and the amount of insulin according to the changes in your meal and exercise schedules and the carbohydrate content in your food. Insulin lispro, aspart, or glulisine covers each meal. NPH in the morning provides low-level background insulin during the day, and when taken at bedtime, it controls fasting blood sugar the next morning. Insulin action in this plan will look as shown in the following graph.			

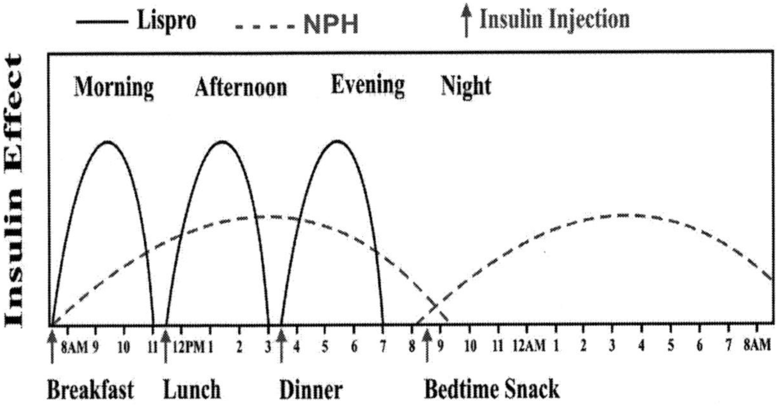

Insulin Plan 4			
Before Breakfast	*Before Lunch*	*Before Dinner*	*Before Bedtime*
Intermediate-acting NPH **plus** short-acting regular	Short-acting regular	Short-acting regular	Intermediate-acting NPH
This is a variation of plan 3. It uses short-acting regular insulin in place of rapid acting lispro, aspart, or glulisine. The action of regular insulin in each injection in this plan will look as shown in the graph below.			

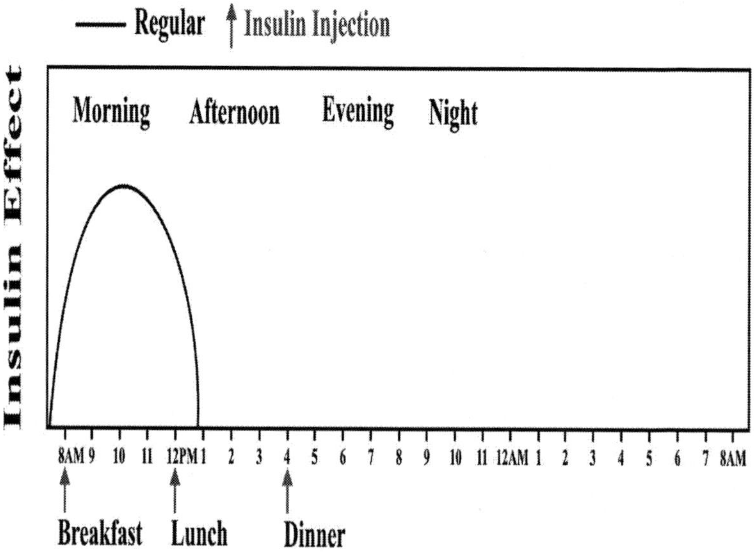

Insulin Plan 5			
Before Breakfast	*Before Lunch*	*Before Dinner*	*Before Bedtime*
Long-acting glargine or detemir **plus** rapid-acting lispro, aspart or glulisine	Rapid-acting lispro, aspart or glulisine	Rapid-acting lispro, aspart or glulisine	–
This plan is another variation of intensive insulin therapy in plan 3. It uses long-acting in place of the intermediate-acting insulin for providing background insulin. Insulin action of long-acting glargine or detemir in this plan will look as shown in the graph below.			

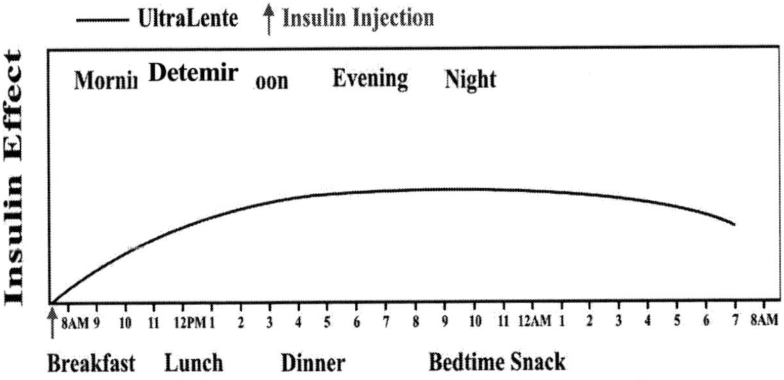

12.3

Insulin Therapy for Type 2 Diabetes

Raised blood sugar, over time, impairs insulin secretion and insulin action in people with type 2 diabetes. As a result, a stage comes when nutrition, exercise, and diabetes pills all fail to control blood sugar in these people. This is the stage when insulin therapy has to be added to control blood sugar. In type 2 diabetes, you usually continue taking diabetes pills along with insulin because these pills help you overcome insulin resistance, a typical feature of type 2 diabetes. Once your blood sugar is well controlled by adding insulin in your treatment plan (and your insulin producing cells have not been totally exhausted), it may be possible to switch back to nutrition, exercise, and diabetes pills to keep blood sugar under control.

Various options of insulin therapy are available in type 2 diabetes. Your doctor, for example, may advise you to take diabetes pills in the day and a small dose of intermediate-acting insulin at bedtime. Injecting insulin at bedtime will prevent your liver from releasing sugar from its stored reserves while you are sleeping, and help you achieve normal fasting blood sugar in the morning. Another but a more advanced option may be to take a reasonable dose of intermediate-acting insulin in the morning, a smaller dose at night, and diabetes pills (metformin or whatever the doctor prescribes) in between. As type 2 diabetes grows chronic, insulin therapy may be gradually intensified, and people with type 2 diabetes may have to follow the same intensified insulin treatment plans as are followed by people with type 1 diabetes. Among the various insulin therapy options for type 2 diabetes, here are four plans:

Insulin Plan 1.1			
Before Breakfast	*Before Lunch*	*Before Dinner*	*Before Bedtime*
–	–	–	Intermediate-acting NPH
This is the start of insulin therapy in people with type 2 diabetes. In addition to diabetes pills, intermediate-acting insulin is added. NPH taken at bedtime suppresses release of sugar from the liver during the night, and lowers fasting blood sugar in the morning.			

Insulin Plan 1. 2			
Before Breakfast	*Before Lunch*	*Before Dinner*	*Before Bedtime*
Intermediate-acting NPH	–	–	–
NPH taken in the morning provides background insulin during the day. This insulin plan, when added to diabetes pills, helps achieve improved control of blood sugar.			

Insulin Plan 1. 3			
Before Breakfast	*Before Lunch*	*Before Dinner*	*Before Bedtime*
Intermediate-acting NPH **plus** short-acting regular	–	–	–

People with type 2 diabetes continue taking diabetes pills and add this insulin plan for better control of their blood sugar. In this plan, regular insulin taken before breakfast assists in overcoming insulin resistance, a condition usually strong in the morning in type 2 diabetes. NPH taken in the morning provides basal or background insulin during the day that helps stabilize blood sugar.

Insulin Plan 1.4			
Before Breakfast	*Before Lunch*	*Before Dinner*	*Before Bedtime*
Intermediate-acting NPH **plus** short-acting regular	–	Intermediate-acting NPH **plus** short-acting regular	–

When one time dosing of insulin (added to diabetes pills) fails to control blood sugar in people with type 2 diabetes, insulin therapy is intensified. In addition to taking diabetes pills, people with type 2 diabetes add this insulin plan for better control of blood sugar. In this plan, regular insulin taken before breakfast assists in overcoming insulin resistance in the morning. NPH taken in the morning provides basal or background insulin during the day. Regular insulin injected in the evening covers dinner, and NPH at dinner helps control fasting blood sugar the next morning.

12.4

Insulin Therapy for Gestational Diabetes

Sometimes diabetes occurs only in pregnancy, a condition called gestational diabetes. Studies suggest that hormonal changes in the body during pregnancy tend to raise blood sugar in about 4 percent of pregnant women.

When lifestyle measures, including healthy eating and regular exercise, fail to reduce raised blood sugar in gestational diabetes, insulin therapy is added. (Generally, the use of diabetes pills is not considered safe during pregnancy.) Insulin therapy, added to healthy eating, improves blood sugar control. Blood sugar improvement reduces the risk for diabetes- related complications in pregnancy, and helps achieve safe deliveries.

Insulin treatment of gestational diabetes has several options, including the use of an insulin pump. The right option will depend on the individual requirements of a patient to be determined by the doctor. One simple option, however, is to take insulin injections twice daily to control diabetes in pregnancy (see table next page). Tip: Short-acting regular insulin is used to control gestational diabetes; rapid-acting insulin, due to its fast action and the associated risk of low blood sugar, is not recommended.

Gestational diabetes usually ends after the pregnancy is over and blood sugar becomes normal. But chances are that after you have had gestational diabetes, you may develop type 2 diabetes later in your life. Maintain healthy weight, eat healthy, and exercise regularly to reduce your risk for developing diabetes in the future. Watch your blood sugar and get it tested periodically to make sure that diabetes does not take you by surprise.

Twice Daily Insulin Injections in Pregnancy			
Time	*Type of Insulin*	*Insulin Ratio*	*Dose*
Before Breakfast	Intermediate-acting NPH Plus Short-acting regular	NPH/regular 2:1	2/3rd of the total dose
Before Dinner	Intermediate-acting NPH Plus Short-acting regular	NPH/regular 1:1	1/3rd of the total dose

In this plan, regular insulin taken before breakfast will help overcome insulin resistance in the morning. NPH will provide background insulin during the day. Regular insulin in the evening will cover dinner, and NPH in this combination will help stabilize fasting blood sugar the next morning.

When pregnancy is over, the body's enhanced need for insulin also ends. After delivery, your body's requirement for insulin returns to its original level before pregnancy. Decrease your insulin dose after delivery to prevent low blood sugar.

12.5

Carbohydrate Counting

Carbohydrate is the main food nutrient that has the maximum impact on raising blood sugar. Carbohydrate containing foods include starches, breads, vegetables, fruits, milk products, and sugars.

To achieve a good control of blood sugar, some people with diabetes who take insulin count the grams of carbohydrates in their meals, and adjust their insulin injection dose directly in proportion to the amount of carbohydrates they eat. This means that when they eat food with an increased or decreased carbohydrate content, they will increase or decrease the dose of insulin. People who do not use insulin, but control blood sugar through diet, exercise, and diabetes pills, can also try to control their blood sugar by increasing or decreasing their carbohydrate intake.

USING CARBOHYDRATE COUNTING

Consult a dietitian how to put the carbohydrate counting into practice. However, several steps are taken to use carbohydrate counting in meal planning:

- First, identify how many calories do you need daily. Assume, you need 2,000 calories per day.
- Second, determine your daily requirement of carbohydrates. Assume that you need to derive 55 percent of your total calories from carbohydrates. Multiplying 2,000 calories by 55%, you get 1,100, which is the number of calories that you should derive from carbohydrate-

containing foods in a day. Because carbohydrates are measured in grams and 1 gram of carbohydrate contains 4 calories, divide 1,100 calories by 4 to get the amount in grams. You get 275 grams, which is your daily carbohydrate requirement in the present example.

- Third, identify the carbohydrate-containing foods and the amount of carbohydrate these foods provide per serving. (Exchange lists available with a dietitian and Nutrition Facts labels on food packages are good sources of determining the carbohydrate values of many foods.)
- Next, spread out your carbohydrate choices over various meals and snacks throughout the day. Your daily eating pattern may include a breakfast, a snack, lunch, then a snack, dinner, and finally, a snack.

CARBOHYDRATE-TO-INSULIN RATIO

The relationship between the amount of carbohydrates you eat and the amount of insulin you inject is called the carbohydrate-to-insulin ratio. There is, however, no standard formula that can determine exactly how many units of injected insulin will cover how many grams of carbohydrates. This is because carbohydrates may be absorbed quickly or slowly into your blood and, therefore, the need for insulin may vary. The time the carbohydrates take to be absorbed as sugar in the blood depends on several factors: the amount of fiber, fat, and protein present in your meals; your physical activity; and the amount of medication circulating in your blood.

Determining the Carbohydrate-to-Insulin Ratio

Although not exact, you can have a fair idea of your carbohydrate-to-insulin ratio after careful monitoring in which you and a dietitian will work together. You will keep records for at least 2 weeks of the carbohydrates you have eaten, the units of insulin you have injected, and self-monitored results of your blood sugar. Only after you achieve your blood sugar target by a specific amount of insulin, your carbohydrate-to-insulin ratio can be determined.

Many people, however, may find from their experience that they need roughly 1 unit of regular insulin to cover 15 grams of carbohydrates (such as 1 slice of bread or 1 small orange). Therefore, when these people eat a meal containing 75 grams of carbohydrates, for example, they will inject 75/15= 5 units of regular insulin to cover the after-meal rise of blood sugar. Note, however, that this is a mere estimate and may differ from person to person and be different in varying situations.

13

Treating Diabetes in Children

Children may have type 1 or type 2 diabetes. Type 1 diabetes is typically a disease of childhood and can appear in children at any age. Its highest incidence, however, is in children 10 to 14 years old. In recent years, the onset of type 1 diabetes in children younger than 5 years has also increased. Recently, type 2 diabetes, typically a disease of adults, has also been occurring in children in alarming proportions.

In general, the principles of diabetes care that are relevant to adults are also applicable to children with diabetes. There are, however, certain aspects of diabetes care that are either unique or have a greater relevance for children.

BLOOD SUGAR GOALS

Strict control of blood sugar is not desirable in infants, because it heightens their risk for low blood sugar. Frequent episodes of low blood sugar are harmful to infants because at this age they are undergoing rapid physical and mental development, and low blood sugar can damage their growth. As children grow older and by the time they become adolescents, sufficient brain development has already occurred. Low blood sugar episodes at this age will not usually be damaging to the brain. However, as children with diabetes grow older, their risk for diabetes complications tends to increase. This is the reason that blood sugar goals for children 13 to 19 years old are more demanding than those of younger children. The following table lists desirable blood sugar goals for children with diabetes.

Blood Sugar Goals for Children with Diabetes		
Child's Age	*Before Meals Blood Sugar**	*Bedtime/OverNight Blood Sugar**
Less than 6 years	100 to 180 mg dL (5.6 to 18 mmol/L)	110 to 200 mg/dL (6.1 to 11.1 mmol/L)
6 to 12 years (School children)	90 to 180 mg/dL (5.0 to 18 mmol/L)	100 to 180 mg/dL (5.6 to 18 mmol/L)
13 to 19 years (Adolescents and young adults)	90 to 130 mg/dL (5.0 to 7.2 mmol/L)	90 to 150 mg/dL (5.0 to 8.3 mmol/L)
* Plasma blood values (laboratory referenced).		
Source: Adapted from American Diabetes Association. "Position Statement. Standards of Medical Care in Diabetes.2007." *Diabetes Care*, vol.30 (suppl.1) (2007).		

TREATING TYPE 1 DIABETES IN CHILDREN

Treatment of type 1 diabetes requires administration of insulin to control blood sugar. The insulin treatment has to be highly individualized according to the insulin needs and typical conditions of your child:

- Infants with diabetes require very small amounts of insulin. The regular insulin of U-100 strength is diluted into U-50, U-25, or U-10 strengths. To dilute insulin, use the diluting solution provided by the manufacturing company.

- As your child grows older, his or her insulin needs will increase as noted before. How much insulin does your child with diabetes need is to be determined by the doctor. The total daily insulin dose of a young child, for example, may be 0.5 unit per 1 kg of body weight of the child. The dose may be distributed between two meals as indicated in the table below.

Two-Injection Insulin Plan for A Child with Type 1 Diabetes		
Time of Injection- 30 Minutes before:	*Type of Insulin*	*Dose*
Breakfast	Intermediate-acting (NPH) Plus short-acting regular with NPH/regular ratio of 2:1	2/3 of the daily dose calculated at 0.5 unit of insulin per 1 kg of body weight
Dinner	Same as above	1/3 of the daily dose calculated at 0.5 unit of insulin per 1 kg of body weight

- This requirement will increase as the child grows and becomes a school-age child. At this age, he or she may need 1.0 unit of insulin per 1 kg of body weight, per day.
- Because growing age and puberty are associated with

insulin resistance, growing adolescents need a greater amount of insulin. At this stage, they may need 1.0 to 1.5 units of insulin per 1 kg of body weight per day to fight back insulin resistance and to control blood sugar. Since the insulin need of a child changes with the passage of time, it is necessary that the doctor periodically reassesses the insulin requirement of your child.

- As children grow older and reach adolescence, their lifestyles tend to be hectic and their meal times become irregular. In such settings, fixed doses of insulin at consistently the same time every day will not be appropriate. It is better to build insulin plans around their meals. This means that children with diabetes should take insulin when they eat their meals and not at fixed times of the day. To build such a plan, there can be various options of insulin combinations. One option is to devise an insulin plan in which your adolescent receives a long-acting insulin such as insulin glargine or detemir in the morning, and the short-acting regular or rapid-acting insulin —lispro, aspart, or glulisine— before each meal (see insulin plans 3 to 5 in title 12.2). Such treatment plans will provide increased flexibility of lifestyle to the adolescent, while achieving good control of blood sugar at the same time.

TREATING TYPE 2 DIABETES

Unless a child diagnosed with type 2 diabetes presents such critical medical conditions as increased acids in the blood or extremely high blood sugar (conditions that require insulin therapy right away), children with type 2 diabetes are treated in almost the same way as adults with this disease are treated:

- First, try lifestyle measures such as weight reduction, increased physical activity, and healthy eating.

- When lifestyle modification is not enough to control blood sugar, the doctor may add diabetes pills to the treatment plan.
- To treat children with type 2 diabetes, diabetes pills of the metformin class may be used first for two main reasons. Metformin, unlike sulfonylurea, does not raise the risk of low blood sugar, and second, it helps reduce weight in obese and overweight children.
- When metformin added to lifestyle modification fails to control blood sugar, diabetes pills of the sulfonylurea class may be added.
- Diabetes pills of another class — meglitinide—may be especially useful for adolescents whose meal times are irregular. This medicine is quick in controlling raised blood sugar after eating.Taking these pills just before meals helps control the after-meal rise of blood sugar.
- Because diabetes pills of the troglitazone class have been linked to liver failure, use of these pills is not recommended in children.
- If combination therapy, consisting of different classes of diabetes pills, fails to control your child's blood sugar, insulin therapy may be added. Insulin treatment may be started by administering insulin injection once or twice daily. (See insulin treatment plans in title 12.3.)
- When diabetes becomes chronic, and blood sugar control is lost, the doctor may advise to discontinue the use of diabetes pills, and start full-fledged insulin therapy.

14

Pancreas Transplantation

Pancreas transplantation is a major form of surgery, which is increasingly becoming a standard treatment for extreme cases of uncontrolled diabetes, especially type 1. This surgery aims to "cure" diabetes, prevent, and in some cases, even reverse diabetes complications. Pancreas transplantation is usually considered in people having diabetes for more than 20 years.

Beta cells of the pancreas excrete insulin that controls blood sugar and keeps it within the normal range. In type 1 diabetes, beta cells are destroyed and people with this disease must inject insulin to control blood sugar. Some people, however, may fail to control their blood sugar despite intensive insulin therapy in which they take multiple insulin injections every day, or use an insulin pump for continuous infusion of insulin day and night. These people face recurring situations in which their blood sugar either rises too high or falls too low.

Over time, high blood sugar tends to cause long-term complications such as sight loss, kidney failure, amputation, heart attack, stroke, and nerve damage. Extremely low levels of blood sugar, on the other hand, can cause stroke or even death. The situation becomes all the more dangerous when, due to nerve damage from long-standing diabetes, people develop low blood sugar unawareness in which they even fail to recognize the symptoms of low blood sugar. In such a condition, these people are unable to treat low blood sugar in time, and may end up in a medical emergency.

When intensive insulin therapy totally fails to control diabetes, pancreas transplantation may become a desirable option for people exposed to excessive risk of diabetes complications. After pancreas transplantation, beta cells of the transplanted pancreas start secreting insulin, and blood sugar control is restored.

TYPES OF PANCREAS TRANSPLANT

Pancreas transplantations are of three kinds:

Whole Pancreas Transplant

In this procedure, a whole pancreas extracted from a person who has just died (cadaver donor), is transplanted into the recipient.

Segmented Pancreas Transplant

In segmented pancreas transplantation, a portion, usually half of the pancreas of a living donor, is separated through an operation and transplanted in the recipient. The donor may be a relative or a person whose pancreas tissues match with those of the recipient.

Islet Cells Transplant

Islets of Langerhans, which contain insulin-producing beta cells, are isolated from the pancreas of a person who has just died. These islets are injected into the liver (instead of the pancreas) of the recipient because it is easier to reach the liver through its wide portal vein. The islets start manufacturing and secreting insulin in the liver, from where it directly enters the bloodstream and starts controlling blood sugar. However, beta cells injected into the liver take some time before they develop blood supply and start secreting insulin. Until such time as the beta cells start working, the recipient receives insulin injections to control blood sugar.

Islet cell transplantation is carried out under local anesthesia; the procedure is finished in less than 60 minutes; and it is less invasive than the transplantation of a whole or segmented pancreas. Islet cell transplants, like other organ transplants, require a lifelong use of anti-rejection drugs called the immunosuppressants. These drugs help prevent the body from rejecting the transplanted islet cells. The anti-rejection drugs, however, may cause certain side effects such as reduction in kidney function, infections, and raised blood cholesterol levels.

FORMS OF PANCREAS TRANSPLANT

Pancreas transplantation can take any of the following three forms:

Simultaneous Pancreas-Kidney Transplant (SPK)

People who have uncontrolled diabetes and have developed kidney failure may have a procedure in which the pancreas and kidney are transplanted simultaneously in one surgery. SPK makes people become independent of insulin injections and free from the need of dialysis. If the surgery involving the pancreas-kidney transplant is too extensive or risky for some people because of their specific health conditions, islet cell transplant being a less invasive procedure, may be considered with a kidney transplant.

Pancreas After Kidney Transplant (PAK)

A person whose kidneys have failed and whose pancreas also does not work may need transplantation of both the organs. In PAK, the patient first receives a kidney transplant when the kidney is available from a living donor. Later, when the pancreas available from a living donor. Later, when the pancreas or islets are available from a deceased donor, the patient receives the pancreas or islet transplant.

Pancreas Transplant Alone (PTA)

In a few patients, the pancreas is transplanted alone without combining a kidney transplant.

WHY THE PANCREAS AND KIDNEY TRANSPLANTS ARE COMBINED

A combined pancreas-kidney transplant is done for two main reasons:

First, kidney failure is a common long-term complication of uncontrolled diabetes. When the kidneys fail, the patient has to undergo dialysis regularly to remain alive. Dialysis, however, is an inconvenient and time consuming procedure. A kidney transplant restores the vital kidney functions and frees a person from the need for dialysis.

Second, if blood sugar remains uncontrolled even after kidney transplantation, diabetes continues, damaging the transplanted kidney, leading to kidney failure again. To prevent this risk, the pancreas is also transplanted. The transplanted pancreas controls blood sugar and helps prevent organ failure or organ loss from diabetes. For these reasons, the patient receives a simultaneous pancreas-kidney or a pancreas transplant after the kidney has been transplanted.

WHY THE PANCREAS IS TRANSPLANTED ALONE

Some people with diabetes may not develop diabetic kidney disease, but have serious problems in controlling their blood sugar. These people experience frequent and sudden episodes of very high or very low blood sugar. Both these conditions may lead to severe long-term complications and can cause death. To reduce these risks and control diabetes, a pancreas-alone transplant may be considered.

WHO IS A CANDIDATE FOR PANCREAS TRANSPLANT

Those who are likely to be most benefited from receiving a pancreas transplant include:

- People with type 1 diabetes whose bodies do not produce insulin and who have lost control over their diabetes. These people are unable to control their blood sugar despite intensive insulin therapy, and are at increased risk of organ damage and organ failure due to diabetes. People with type 2 diabetes are not usually considered for pancreas transplant, because their bodies still produce some insulin. However, a review about transplantation published in the *Diabetes Care* in 2005 observed that the type of diabetes is an irrelevant factor in deciding who should receive a pancreas transplant. The review suggested that people with type 1 or type 2 diabetes, older than 50 years, who are unable to control their blood sugar, and who are not obese at the time of transplantation, may be the right candidates for pancreas transplantation.
- People with type 1 and type 2 diabetes who need kidney transplantation. The pancreas transplant with a kidney transplant will help control blood sugar, and prevent failure of the transplanted kidney from diabetes.
- Individuals who experience frequent, sudden swings of very low or very high blood sugar, or who go through frequent episodes of ketoacidosis in which blood acids become very high.

- People with diabetes who have developed a severe form of low blood sugar unawareness. In such a condition, these people fail to recognize the symptoms of low blood sugar. This situation, when left untreated, can lead to coma or death.

14.1

More on Pancreas Transplantation

Generally, pancreas or islet transplantation, when successful, controls blood sugar and improves the quality of life in people with diabetes. Reasons:

- Transplanted pancreas leads to regular secretion of natural insulin that effectively controls blood sugar.
- It eliminates the severe dietary restrictions needed to control blood sugar.
- It ends the need for insulin injections or an insulin pump. People who injected insulin before pancreas transplantation gain insulin independence after the pancreas is transplanted.
- Hemoglobin A1C levels become normal after pancreas transplantation. In many transplant recipients, the A1C level decreased from 9.4 to 5.5 percent, a remarkable reduction that shows an excellent control of blood sugar. The transplantation in these people also led to improvement in their nerve damage, albumin excretion, high blood pressure, LDL cholesterol, and diabetic eye damage.
- It ends the need for frequent monitoring of blood sugar.
- It prevents diabetes emergencies such as blood sugar rising too high or becoming too low, or the acids increasing too much in the blood (ketoacidosis).
- The simultaneous pancreas-kidney transplant helps prevent the development of diabetic kidney disease.

LIMITATIONS OF PANCREAS TRANSPLANTATION

All types of pancreas transplants have limitations:

- Pancreas transplantation is a major surgery, and like other major surgeries, is associated with the risk of sudden death.
- Although an islet transplant involves less invasive surgery than other kinds of pancreas transplants, this procedure has generally been less successful in controlling blood sugar. However, some advances have been made recently in islet transplantation.
- Pancreas transplants do not reverse certain long-term complications of diabetes in advanced stages. Diabetic eye disease in its advanced stage, or heart diseases caused by diabetes, are not reversed by the pancreas transplant. The transplantation, though, is partly successful in reversing long-term nerve damage and kidney damage.
- Pancreas-alone transplants are less successful than the simultaneous pancreas-kidney transplants (SPKs).
- Some people with diabetes who receive pancreas transplants become free from insulin injections, and their blood sugar remains under control for years. However, sooner or later, diabetes tends to reoccur in most people after implantation, and ultimately, they have to restart taking insulin injections. This risk is especially significant in people with greater age and body weight at the time they receive a pancreas implant.
- The main disadvantage of pancreas transplantation is the use of powerful anti-rejection drugs for preventing the body from rejecting the transplanted pancreas. While these drugs help prevent rejection of the transplant, they

impair the body's infection-fighting system, resulting in increased risk for infections and cancers. However, now the preventive use of comparatively safe antiviral drugs, has significantly reduced the risk of such infections after organ transplantation.

- Also, the anti-rejection drugs used after transplantation not only reduce the action of insulin, but also increase insulin resistance in the body. As a result, many recipients of the pancreas transplants fail to achieve complete insulin independence and again they have to take insulin injections.

IMPORTANCE OF DIET AND EXERCISE

A healthy diet and low-impact exercises are important after the transplantation. A healthy diet such as suggested in title 1 will help reduce the side effects of powerful anti-rejection drugs that the patient has to take regularly after receiving the transplant. Physical fitness, in general, improves quality of life and is equally beneficial after the transplantation. Regular exercise improves blood circulation, elevates mood, and increases stamina and strength.

SUCCESS RATE OF PANCREAS TRANSPLANTATION

Development in surgical procedures has raised the success rates of pancreas transplantation. According to a report of the United Network of Organ Sharing, more than 83 percent of the people who received pancreas-kidney transplants, and more than 76 percent of the people who received pancreas-alone transplants achieved insulin independence 1 year of transplantation. At present, the simultaneous pancreas-kidney transplant (SPK) is the most common and preferred procedure among all the forms of pancreas transplants; it has a better rate of survival and success.

According to the data base of the Organ Procurement and Transplantation Network, more than 5, 900 pancreas-alone transplants, and more than 15, 300 kidney-pancreas transplants were performed in the United States from January 1988 to September 2008. The national patient waiting list for organ transplants maintained by the United Network of Organ Sharing shows about 4,000 patients waiting for pancreas and pancreas-kidney transplants as in September 2008. However, a short supply of donors' pancreases and the administration of powerful anti-rejection drugs, having serious side effects, are the main hurdles in the the way of these operations.

In Edmonton, Canada, scientists successfully experimented with a new method of islet transplantation called Edmonton Protocol. Islet cell transplants, using this protocol, have been remarkably successful in reversing type 1 diabetes in all the recipients. Edmonton protocol of islet cell transplantation uses an improved technique to isolate islet cells from the pancreas of a deceased donor. This technique transplants fresh instead of frozen islets used in the earlier procedures; it transplants a large number of islets (islet cells from two to three donor pancreases for one transplant) to improve the chances of their survival; and it uses improved anti-rejection drugs after transplantation.

Scientists in the United States are extensively researching islet cell transplantation, using the Edmonton technique. If the technique proves successful on a large scale, and safe in the long term, islet cell transplantation may become the standard treatment for type 1 diabetes. To solve the problem of shortage of islet cells for transplantation, experiments are being done to use the islet cells from pigs, transplant a person's own stem cells (a kind of neutral or unspecialized cells in the body), and develop artificial beta cells in the laboratories.

Appendix

BMI Chart

Height (inches)	Your weight in pounds								
58	110	115	119	124	129	134	138	143	148
59	114	119	124	128	133	138	143	148	153
60	118	123	128	133	138	143	148	153	158
61	122	127	132	137	143	148	153	158	164
62	126	131	136	142	147	153	158	164	169
63	130	135	141	146	152	158	163	169	175
64	134	140	145	151	157	163	169	174	180
65	138	144	150	156	162	168	174	180	186
66	142	148	155	161	167	173	179	186	192
67	146	153	159	166	172	178	185	191	198
68	151	158	164	171	177	184	190	197	203
69	155	162	169	176	182	189	196	203	209
70	160	167	174	181	188	195	202	209	216
71	165	172	179	186	193	200	208	215	222
72	169	177	184	191	199	206	213	221	228
73	174	182	189	197	204	212	219	227	235
74	179	186	194	202	210	218	225	233	241
75	184	192	200	208	216	224	232	240	248
76	189	197	205	213	221	230	238	246	254
77	194	203	211	220	228	237	245	254	262
BMI	**23**	**24**	**25**	**26**	**27**	**28**	**29**	**30**	**31**

Look for your height in the "Height" column. Move across the table until you find your weight. The 2-digit number at the bottom of the column is your BMI. A BMI of less than 25 represents healthy weight; 25 or higher is overweight; and 30 or higher is obesity.

Source: Adapted from NIH/National Heart, Lung, and Blood Institute.

Selected References

American College of Endocrinology. *Pocket Guide to Management of Type 2 Diabetes.* 2004

American Diabetes Association. "Standards of Medical Care in Diabetes-2008."*Diabetes Care*, vol. 31(2008).

——."Pancreas and Islet Transplantation in Type 1 Diabetes. Position Statement." *Diabetes Care*, vol. 29(2006).

American Heart Association, Inc. "NCEP Report: Implications of Recent Clinical Trials for the National Cholesterol Education Program Adult Treatment Panel III Guidelines." *Circulation*, vol.110 (2004).

Anderson, J.H., and others. Multicenter Insulin Lispro Study Group. "Mealtime Treatment with Insulin Analog Improves Postprandial Hyperglycemia and Hypoglycemia in Patients with Non-insulin-Dependent Diabetes Mellitus." *Archives of Internal Medicine*, vol.157(11) (1997).

Apidra Injection [*package Insert*]. November 2005.

Bell, D.S., and F. Ovalle. "Long-Term Efficacy of Triple Oral Therapy for Type 2 Diabetes Mellitus." *Endocrine Practice*, vol. 8 (2002).

Bergenstal, R.M., and Gavin JR III. "The Role of Self-Monitoring of Blood Sugar in the Care of Peole with Diabetes: Report of a Global Consensus Conference." *American Jounal of Medicine*, vol. 118 (suppl. A) (2005).

Buchanan, T.A., and others. "Preservation of Pancreatic Beta-Cell Function and Prevention of Type 2 Diabetes by Pharmacological Treatment of Insulin Resistance in High-Risk Hispanic Women. *Diabetes,* vol. 51(2002).

Byetta (exenatide) Injection [*package Insert*]. 2005.

Byetta [*Package Insert*]. 2007.

Davidson, J.A., and A. Wilkinson. "The International Expert Panel on New-Onset Diabetes After Transplantation: New-Onset Diabetes After Transplantation 2003 International Consensus Guidelines: An Endocrinogist's View." *Diabetes Care*, vol. 27 (2004).

Denke, M.A. "Cholesterol-Lowering Diets: A Review of the Evidence." *Archives of Internal Medicine*, vol. 155 (1995).

Diabetes Control and Complications Trial Research Group. "The Effect of Intensive Treatment of Diabetes on the Development and Progression of Long-Term Complicationsin Insulin-Dependent Diabetes Mellitus." *New England Journal of Medicine*, vol. 329 (1993).

Epocrates, Inc. *Epocrates Drug Reference*. 2007.

Evans, Josie M.M., and others. "Frequency of Blood Glucose Monitoring in Relation to Glycaemic Control: Observational Study with Diabetes Database." *British Medical Journal*, vol. 319 (1999).

Exubera Inhaler [*package Insert*]. 2006.

Farkas-Hirsch, R., ed. American Diabetes Association. "Insulin Infusion Pump Therapy." *Intensive Diabetes Management.* 1995.

Fass, A., and others. "The Efficacy of Self-Monitoring of Blood Glucose in NIDDM Subjects."*Diabetes Care*, vol. 20 (1997).

Gallichan, M. "Self-Monitoring of Blood Glucose by People with Diabetes: Evidence Based Practice." *British Medical Journal*, vol. 314 (1997).

Haslet, Christopher, and others, eds. *Davidson's Principles and Practice of Medicine*. 19th ed. 2002.

Hebel, S.K., ed. *Drug Facts and Comparisons*. 1998.

Hirsch, I.B. "Drug Therapy: Insulin Analogues." *New Engl Journal of Medicine*, vol. 352(2) (2005).

Hirsch, I.B., and others. "A Real-World Approach to Insulin Therapy in Primary Care Practice." *Clinical Diabetes*, vol. 23(2005).

Humalog [*Package Insert*]. 2004.

J anuvia (sitagliptin phosphate) [Package Insert]. 006.

Johansen, K. "Efficacy of Metformin in the Treatment of NIDDM." *Diabetes Care*, vol. 22 (1999).

Lantus [*Package Insert*]. 2006.

Levemir injection [*Package insert*]. 2005.

Lindstorm, T., and others. "Long-term Improvement of Glycemic Control by Insulin Treatment in NIDDM Patients with Secondary Failure." *Diabetes Care*, vol. 17 (1994).

Martin, S., and others. "Self-monitoring of Blood Glucose in Type 2 Diabetes and Long-Term Outcome: An Epidemiological Cohort Study." *Diabetologia*, vol.49(2006).

McEvoy., G.E. American Society of Health-System Pharmacists. "Insulins General Statement." *American Hospital Formulary Service Drug Information*. 2005.

Medical Economics Company. *Physicians' Desk Reference*. 56th ed. 2002.

Mecklenburg, R.S., and others. "Long-Term Metabolic Control with Insulin Pump Therapy." *New England Journal of Medicine*, vol. 313 (1985).

Moreland, E.C., and others. "Use of a Blood Glucose Monitoring Manual to Enhance Monitoring Adherence in Adults with Diabetes: A randomized Controlled Trial." *Archives of Internal Medicine*, vol.166 (2006).

Mudaliar, S., and R.R.Henry. "New Oral Therapies for Type 2 Diabetes Mellitus: The Glitazones or Insulin Sensitizers." *Annual Review of Medicine*, vol. 52 (2001).

National Committee for Clinical Laboratory Standards. *Ancillary (Bedside) Blood Glucose Testing in Acute and Chronic Care Facilities: Approved Guideline.* 1994.

NovoLog [*Package Insert*]. 2005.

O'Brien, T., and others. "Hyperlipidemia and Diabetes Mellitus." *Mayo Clinic Proceedings*, vol. 73 (1998).

Pickup J., Keen H. "Continuous Subcutaneous Insulin Infusion at 25 Years: Evidence Base for the Expanding Use of Insulin Pump Therapy in Typc 1 Diabetes." *Diabetes Care*, vol.25 (2002).

Pickup, John C. , and others, eds. *Text Book of Diabetes*. 3rd ed. 2003.

Raskin, P., and others. "Initiating Insulin Therapy In Type 2 Diabetes: A Comparison of Biphasic and Basal Insulin Analogs." *Diabetes Care*, vol. 28(2) 2005.

Robertson, R.P., and others. "Pancreas and Islet Transplantation for Patients with Diabetes Mellitus (Technical Review)." *Diabetes Care*, vol. 23 (2000).

Scheen, A.J., and P.J.Lefebvre. "Oral Diabetic Agents: A Guide to Selection." *Drugs*, vol. 55 (1998).

Snow, V, and others. "Control in the Management of Type 2 Diabetes: A Clical Practice Guidelines from the American College of Physicians."*Annals of Internal Medicine*, vol.140(2004).

Starlix (nateglinide) [*Package Insert*]. 2004.

Stevens, R.B., and others."Is Islet Transplantation a Realistic Therapy for the Treatment of Type 1 Diabetes in the Near Future?" *Clinical Diabetes*, vol. 19 (2) (2001).

Sutherland, D.E. "Pancreas Transplantation as a Treatment for Diabetes: Indications and Outcome." Current Therapy in Endocrinology and Metabolism, vol. 5 (1994)

Symlin [*Medication Guide]*. 2005.

Symlin (pramlintide acetate) Injection [*Package Insert*]. 2005.

"Therapy for the Treatment of Type 1 Diabetes in the Near Future?" *Clinical Diabetes*, vol. 19 (2) (2001).

Wajchenberg, B.L. "Beta-Cell Failure in Diabetes and Preservation by Clinical Treatment." *Endocrine Reviews,* vol. 28 (2007).

Index